THE BODY PLAN PLUS FOOD DIARY

Hello & Welcome

Your Food Diary is divided into two sections.

Section 1

You should read this section first - It's everything you need to know about your new Food Diary. Once you have read this section, you are ready to **Get Started**!

Section 2

Your Food Diary - **Lets Get Started!**

HELLO AND WELCOME

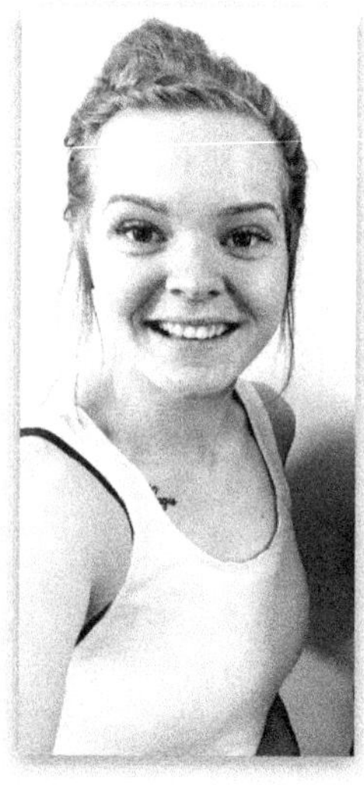

My name is Tania and I'm a certified Personal Trainer. I came into this career path through a personal journey of my own having lost a total of 7 stone.

To start with I tried different diets and various exercise routines - I lost some weight, but I wasn't finding the experience pleasant! I constantly felt tired, hungry, irritable and to be honest generally quite miserable!

After a few more weeks of feeling this way - I quit! Instead I simply said to myself, "Instead of trying to lose weight I will just try not to put more on" I went back to my original eating habits but instead of 3 Pizza's and two litres of pop in a binge, I had to 2 pizza's and 1 litre of pop. And I started to walk a little more instead of driving around all the time.

TIME TO CHECK I WASN'T GAINING WEIGHT ANYMORE!

When I finally plucked up the courage to stand on the scales in hope I hadn't gained more weight - I got quite a shock! I had actually lost half a stone… How was this possible? I was eating Pizza's, Burgers and ready meals galore!   OK… Not as much as I used to, but still it was a pretty poor diet.

I needed to know why I was losing weight. Why was I finding it easy to lose weight now, basically without trying, than when I first started on a dieting plan?

The Penny dropped - It wasn't what I was eating, it was simply the quantity. It was simple maths, there are less Calories in 2 Pizza's than there are in 3… Sounds obvious to me now, but in the beginning , when you have no knowledge of Calories in vs Calories out, you simply think dieting is about eating certain foods!

I wanted to know why I was losing weight without all the original feelings of feeling hungry and miserable. What was I doing right? I researched or should I say "Googled" more and more information about weight loss, activity and fitness and came across BMI Calculators, which simply told me I was still FAT… Not very inspirational and quite depressing!

I started to look up things like Metabolic Rate and Metabolism. It sounds boring but the knowledge put me on a path to losing even more and more weight. While researching Metabolic rate I came across another Weight Loss Calculator - The BMR Calculator - Basal Metabolic Rate. Basically it tells you how many Calories you need per day to Run / Fuel your Body - Based on your current weight and activity.

So in a nutshell -   If you consume the same amount of Calories as your body burns off in any single day - You stay the same weight! More Calories and you gain weight, Less Calories and you lose weight!   OK… You already know this and it may be common sense - **So why is it so hard to lose weight?**

I learnt - And this is the magic part! If you reduce this BMR figure by 300 to 500 Calories, you don't notice the Calorie Reduction - Therefore you don't feel hungry or miserable. And this is what I was feeling… I had found this "**Happy Zone**" by chance. I was reducing my Calorie intake by just the right amount to make me feel happy and content all day long.

If you don't know how many Calories your body needs per day - You can't reduce your Calorie intake by just the right amount for your body to feel happy about it…. This is why Diets fail…!

I wanted to keep my body in the "**Happy Zone**" so I needed to work out a way to "**Keep on top**" of my Calorie Calculations easily.   I wasn't on a short term diet, I wanted to lifestyle change!

I knew exactly how many Calories I needed to feel "**Happy & Content**" but I didn't want to spend all my time looking up the Calorie Content of everything I was eating, so I created my own Food Diary / Organiser.

It was a work in progress and I had to make quite a few changes before I got it just right. Now I know the Calorie content of everything that passes my lips…   I knew my Daily Calorie Goal and I knew the Calorie Content of the foods I enjoy…. As long as I didn't go over my Calorie Goal - I lost weight that day!

Everything became so simple because I just got more organised with my Calories! The more Food Calorie Values I wrote down the easier my calculations became! Soon my Food Diary consisted of a **Calorie Library, Set Menus** and a **Daily Food Tracker,** ensuring I never went over my Daily Calorie Goal.

My Food Diary is here for You to use and Copy my Success!

My Weight Loss Journey was an Education. I wanted to share it all in this Diary, but there simply isn't enough space. So I have some missing pages which contain valuable information and knowledge. These pages are on my website - **Online Extra Content**. Where prompted throughout this Diary, please visit my website to learn more… Knowledge will really help you!

Tania x

ONLINE EXTRA PAGES

There just isn't enough space for it all...!

All the pages that can't fit in this Food Diary can be found on my Website.

www.thebodyplanplus.com

It's an education and everything I learnt. This knowledge made my weight loss Journey a success. I urge you to read it and learn it because it will make you look at weight loss and exercise differently. Motivation to lose weight is one thing, but motivation and knowledge makes it a whole lot easier.

Find the missing pages.

To find the online extra content (Missing Pages) go to my site and select **MORE >** from the menu.

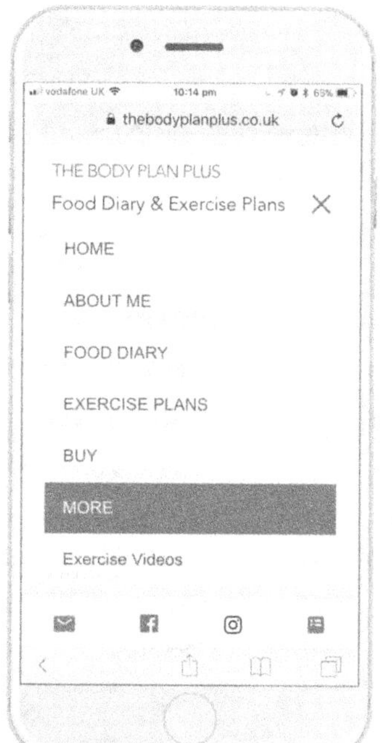

In this section you will find:

- Calorie Goal Calculator
- The Missing Pages
- Exercise Videos
- 10 Weeks to Wow!
- Home Workout Equipment
- Calories Per Gram Calculator
- Quick View Calorie Library
- Easy Set Menus

When you select (The Missing Pages) a list of the content will be displayed, as seen on the opposite page. It's an education, and you will greatly benefit from this knowledge.

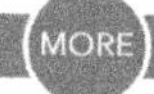

THE MISSING PAGES - IT'S AN EDUCATION!

Dieting

- Magic Formula for Weight Loss
- Keeping it all Fair and Well Balanced
- Calorie Tracking, Extra Benefits

Questions & Answers

- What is the Average Woman Formula?
- Why 500 Calories?
- Why Do Some People Struggle With Dieting?
- What is Starvation Mode?
- Is the Calorie Goal Calculator 100% Accurate?
- How Much Weight Can I Lose?
- Is this Diary More Suited For Larger People?
- Why is this Form of Dieting Not the Main Stream?

Reference

- Energy Balance
- Calories - Maintain, Gain or Lose
- We are all Different
- The Magic Formula
- It went on so it can come off
- Honest Eating
- The Shopping List
- Wonderful Catch 22
- Body Composition Analyser
- **Reference** - Calorie Library Calculations - Calories Per Single Gram

Exercise

- Finding Your Groove
- The Exercise Habit Effect
- Making Exercise Equal & Making Exercise Fair
- An Exercise Plan that is Designed For Everyone

THE MAGIC FORMULA FOR WEIGHT LOSS

Controlling body weight is maths - Calories in against Calories out, and there is a magic formula to getting the balance just right. **"Using this formula you can obtain Your Perfect Daily Calorie Goal".** When using your **Daily Calorie Goal** you can comfortably lose weight without getting all those feelings attributed to being on a Diet Plan - The main one of course, feeling hungry all the time!

Before we continue - Let me assure you, you don't have to be a mathematician to work it all out, in fact you don't have to do any of the calculations at all, and that's because the internet will do it all for you! All you have to do is fill in the blanks - Your Gender, Height, Weight, Age and Activity Level.

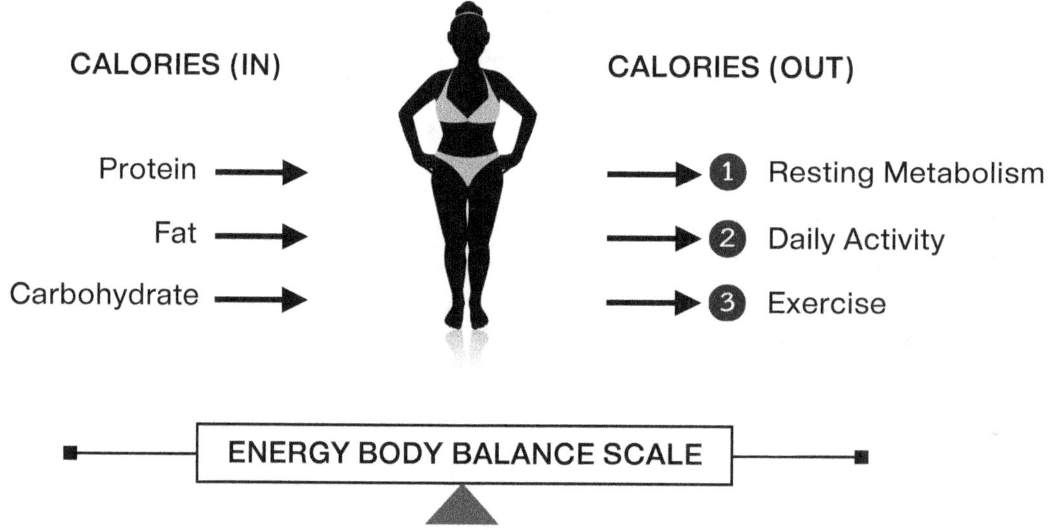

If we get the balance right and you consume the correct amount of Calories (**IN**) for what our body uses up in energy for the day - Calories (**OUT**) then we stay the same weight. To lose weight we simply have to **tip the scales**, and reduce the Calories (**IN**) and or increase the Calories (**OUT**) You can do either or, but a little bit of both is best - **The rule of thumb is 500 Calories!**

Personally I found it easier to play around with between 300 to 500 Calorie Deficit. So when calculating your Calorie Goal you will have the choice.

Why 500 Calories? - For more information go to my website and select **MORE** >

300 - 500 CALORIES IS PART OF THE FORMULA

And You are the Rest!

Our bodies burn Calories (**Energy out**) in three different ways.

1. Calories we burn for just being alive (**This is our Basal Metabolic Rate**)
2. Calories we burn by working, housework, walking, shopping etc - (**Daily Activities**)
3. Calories we burn, by forcing our muscles to work harder then normal (**Exercising**)

And the rate at which we burn the above "3" is **Different For Everyone!**

The energy we use up through the day is mainly determined by our **BODY WEIGHT**, an important figure in the magic formula.

 Important highlighted words - **DIFFERENT FOR EVERYONE & BODY WEIGHT**

Interestingly we burn most of our Calories (**No.1**) for just being alive. This is called your Basal Metabolic Rate.

> Basal Metabolic Rate is the amount of energy expressed in Calories that a person needs to keep the body functioning at rest. Some of those processes are breathing, blood circulation, controlling body temperature, cell growth, brain and nerve function, and contraction of muscles. Basal metabolic rate (**BMR**) affects the rate that a person burns Calories and ultimately whether you maintain, gain, or lose weight. Your Basal Metabolic Rate accounts for about 60 to 75% of the Calories you burn every day.
> The Harris Benedict Equation 1919 (Revised in 1984 & 1990)

 Now we have the formula :-

We simply have to factor **YOU** into the equation to obtain **Your Daily Calorie Goal.**

YOUR DAILY CALORIE GOAL

For the brain boxes among us who would like to see the formula, here it is:-

Step 1 - Calculate Your **BMR (Basal Metabolic Rate)**

Women: BMR = 655 + (4.35 x your weight in pounds) + (4.7 x your height in inches) - (4.7 x age in years)
Men: BMR = 66 + (6.23 x your weight in pounds) + (12.7 x you height in inches) - (6.8 x age in years)

Step 2 - Multiply your **BMR** by the appropriate activity factor, as follows:

- Sedentary (little or no exercise): BMR x 1.2
- Lightly active (light exercise/sports 1-3 days/week): BMR x 1.375
- Moderately active (moderate exercise/sports 3-5 days/week): BMR x 1.55
- Very active (hard exercise/sports 6-7 days a week): BMR x 1.725
- Extra active (very hard exercise/sports & physical job or 2x training): BMR x 1.9

   Super Physical Job - Heavy Labour - Construction - Farm Hand etc

Step 3 - Deduct 300 or 500 Calories for weight loss.

= **Your Personal Daily Calorie Goal!**

Thankfully you don't have to put pen to paper, scratch your head and work it all out. All you have to do is use my online Calorie Goal Calculator

* Is the Calculator 100% Accurate? Go to my website and See **> MISSING PAGES**

ONLINE CALORIE GOAL CALCULATOR

When you have finished reading the rest of this section - Go to my website and select
> MORE and then select **> Calorie Goal Calculator**. Enter your information as required:
Gender - Age - Weight - Height - Exercise Level

Be honest about your Exercise (**PART 3**) as this may impact your results. Saying you do
more exercise than you actually do will result in more Calories being added to your total.

PART 4 Calorie Reduction

Select 300 to 500 for Weight loss and then
hit the "Calculate Calorie Goal" Button

Write Your Maintenance Level &
Calorie Goal here for future Reference.

* Maintenance Level   * Calorie Goal

✱ If you want to stay the same weight use your:

Maintenance Level as Your Daily Calorie Goal

"The amount of Calories you need per day to stay the same weight"

• *Transfer these figures to your Food Diary Page.*

" Remember to Recalculate
Your Calorie Goal Every Time
You Lose 4lb"

MILES BETTER, MORE LOGICAL

So now we know about Energy / Calories (IN), we can all agree that we are different and to lose weight our **Calorie Goal** should be in line and in ratio to our current weight and body structure. Here is an example of 2 real people, Sophie & Helen.

Sophie

Body Weight	11 Stone 2lb
Fat%	34.6%
Fat Mass	24.6 kg
Muscle Mass	44.1 kg
Bone Mass	2.4 kg
BMI	26.9

Weight Loss Goal 1 Stone

Helen

Body Weight	18 Stone 5lb
Fat%	42.2%
Fat Mass	47.1 kg
Muscle Mass	61.3 kg
Bone Mass	3.3 kg
BMI	45.0

Weight Loss Goal 4 Stone

*If we added the activity Calories to each individual, lets say **600 Calories each**, and then subtract their **500 Calorie deficit** for weight loss, the results would look like this:*

BMR	1400		**BMR**	2039
Activity Calories	600		Activity Calories	600
Daily Maintenance	2000		**Daily Maintenance**	2639
Calorie Deficit	500		**Calorie Deficit**	500
Daily Calorie Goal	1500 ✴		Daily Calorie Goal	2139 ✴

> ## 2 VERY DIFFERENT CALORIE GOALS FOR WEIGHT LOSS!
>
> 2 DIFFERENT PEOPLE - 2 VERY DIFFERENT CALORIE GOALS FOR WEIGHT LOSS!
>
> Your **Calorie Goal** should be in line and in ratio to your current weight and structure.

*✴ Data - Two individuals using - Body Composition Analyser - For more info go to my website and select **MORE >***

AND FAIR!

Dieting and slimming clubs offer up some tasty looking healthy "Eats" they are balanced and well thought out.   But a downside to these food plans are, they don't take your Calories (**IN**) & Calories (**OUT**) equation into consideration!   These food plans are **not calculators** and do not know your Daily Calorie Requirement.

Most food plans are structured to supply you with around 1400 - 1500 Calories per day. They base their **Calorie Calculation Information** on the **AVERAGE** Woman equation.

And it goes like this: The Average Woman requires 2000 Calories Per Day - To lose weight reduce this figure by 500 Calories and you get - 1500 Calories - The number most food plans are based on!

Chances are if you're looking to lose weight, you may not be in the average range and therefore it will not supply your body with enough Calories.   Not getting enough Calories for what your body requires, causes your body to do some interesting things - And of course the obvious - Feel hungry!

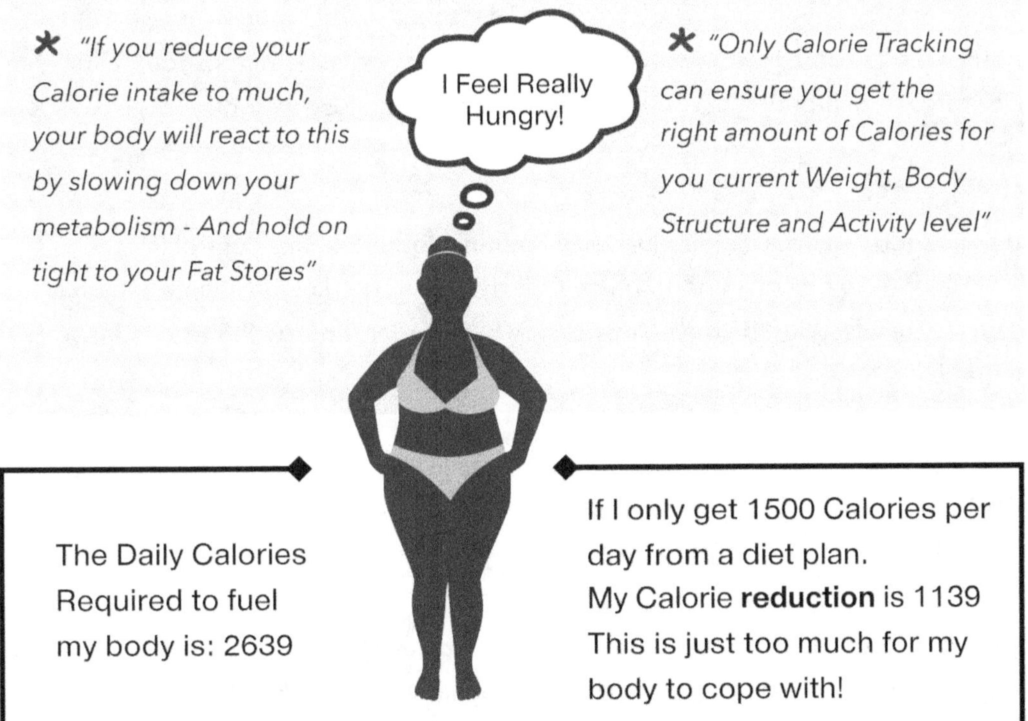

A reduction of **300** to **500** Calories is OK! - **1139 is just way too much!**

TAKE A BREAK - A DIET BREAK!

- **MAINTENANCE**

If we get the balance right, "Calories in" matches or equals "Calories out" you will not gain or lose weight. Or put it another way, if you consume 2500 Calories and burnt off 2500 Calories in a single day, your body stays the same.

- **GAIN**

Sometimes people wish to gain weight, and to do this you would consume more Calories than you burn off in a single day. Or put it another way, if you consume 3000 Calories and burnt off 2000 Calories in a single day, your surplus would be 1000 Calories. Your body has no immediate use for these extra 1000 Calories, so there is only one thing it can do: store them into your body as extra fat or extra muscle.

- **LOSE**

This is the important part if you want to lose weight! If you want to lose weight, then your "Calories in" should be less then your "Calories out".   Or put it another way, if you consume 2000 Calories, and burn off 3000 you will lose weight. You put your body into a "Calorie Deficit". In this case, 1000 calories. These extra 1000 Calories needed to fuel you body have to come from somewhere. So your body gets them from your fat and muscle stores from around your body. So in a nutshell you lose weight.

By definition: Reducing your Calorie intake in "**Dieting Terms**" means controlling the number of Calories to be consumed. These Calories are to be "**Lower**" than what your body needs to fuel itself for the day! Thus calling on your fat "**Energy Stores**" to get you through the day.

So, it does not matter what diet plan or club you have joined or what terminology you use to describe or categorise your foods or food groups - You are controlling your Calories - or put it in another way - Calorie Tracking!

But why guess it? Being on a diet plan that doesn't actually Count Calories, is like trying to run your car without a fuel gauge. And if you don't get enough "**fuel**" - You run out of energy!

Calorie Tracking is the only form of dieting that can be fair and equal for everyone.
It is fair because it's the only method of dieting that allows you to use **YOUR** Daily Calorie
Goal which is unique to you!

If your Daily Calorie Goal is 1900 Calories - Calorie Tracking lets you match it!   And if you
match it - You can actually say "**I Lost Weight Today**"

Diet Bonus!

Now you know your Daily Calorie Goal, you can take a diet break and still not gain
weight. In fact knowing your Calorie Goal allows you to really play around when it comes
food intake control.

To take a diet break, simply add back your "**Reduction Calories**".

For example: If your Calorie Goal is **1900 Calories** add back the Reduction Calories you
choose when using the Online Calculator **300** or **500** Calories.   In this case if you choose
a 500 Calorie Reduction - simply add it back.

1900 + 500 = 2400

2400 Calories would be the new Calorie Goal… YOUR MAINTENANCE LEVEL…!

While consuming your Maintenance level you will not be losing weight, but on the flip
side you will not be gaining weight either.   Not gaining weight is nearly as good as not
losing weight.

Matching your maintenance level gives you a break and also allows your body to be
fooled into thinking - Food is a plenty! This in turn keeps your metabolism running
smoothly.

For more information - Find the (Missing Pages) on my website.

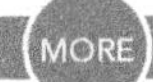

YOUR DIARY - GETTING CALORIE SMART

All of your food related pages start on page 28. You may want to organise yourself a Pen, Pencil, Rubber/Eraser and a couple of Book Marks or Sticky Notes.

These pages are designed to work with each other and full details on how to use them are about to be explained.

Your Diary is organised around four main pages.

- Shopping List
- Calorie Library
- Set Menus
- Food & Daily Calorie Tracker

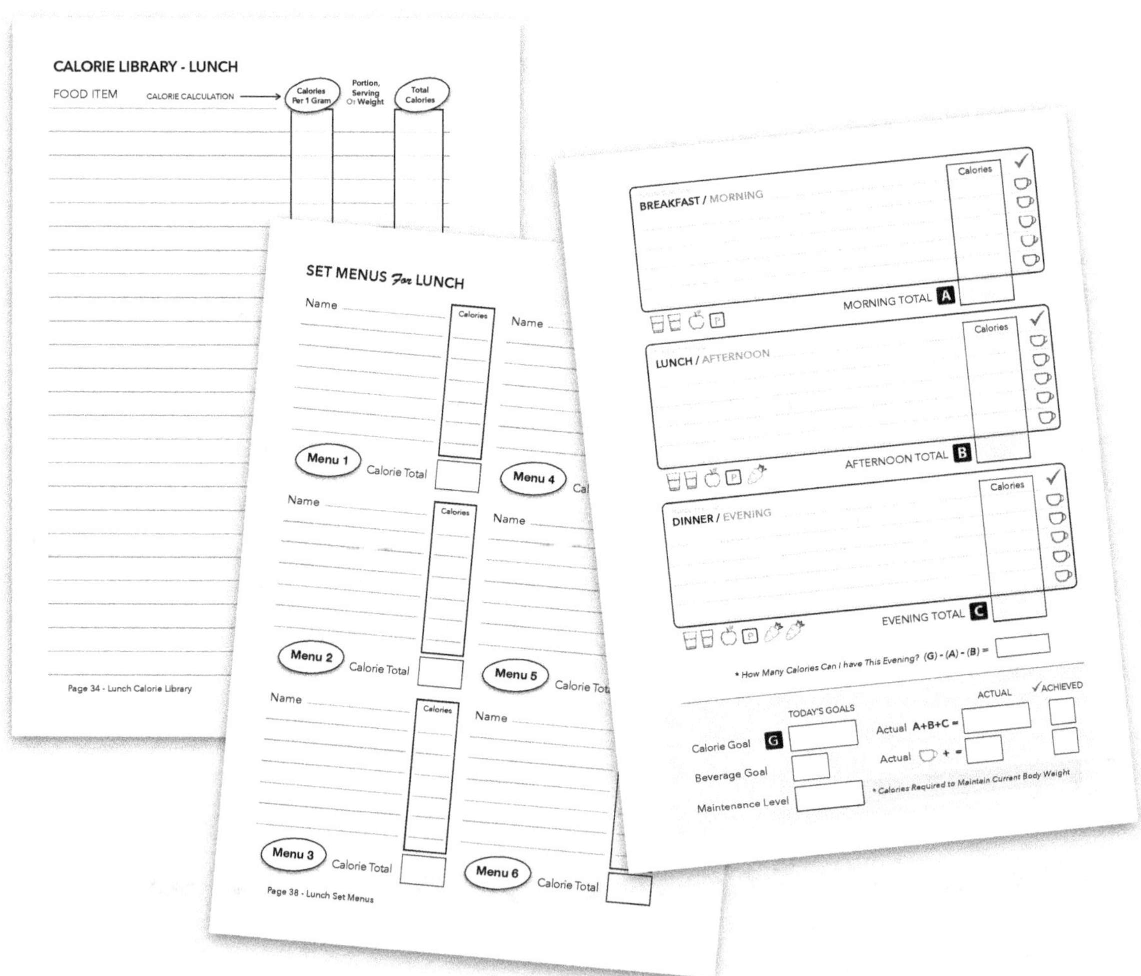

AND FOOD ORGANISED!

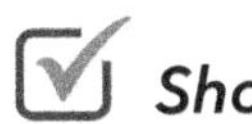 *Shopping List*

The weekly shopping list is very important and will become your guide in purchasing your food for the forthcoming weeks. Don't worry, you will not be making too many changes to begin with but simply becoming slightly more organised. After all, this is not a recipe book, we are talking about honest eating. Handy Hint - Use a pencil, because your shopping list will change.

 *Meal Planner*

Plan the meals that you like and that fit into your lifestyle and family. Meal planning is one of the key elements to successful dieting. If you can crack this, you are half way there. Take some time to think about your Meal Planner sections and you will instantly feel organised and motivated.

 *Calorie Library*

Don't let your Calorie Library confuse you. You do not need to know the Calorie content for every food or each food group, that would by far to much for anyone to know. You only need to know the Calorie content of the foods you eat. It is easier than ever to find out the Calories and values in your food, it's on every tin, packet and box, oh and Google knows the answer!

 *Set Menus*

Fuss free, efficient and super simple. Set menus are really going to make your life diet friendly. Working alongside the shopping list and Meal Planner sections, organising your own Set Menus is going to make recording your food and Calorie values easier than it has ever been!

 *Food & Calorie Tracking*

Your main Diary is laid out over a single page. The workings of this page are explained in greater detail on page 22

YOUR CALORIE LIBRARY

Your **Calorie Library** is one of the key parts to this diary and function. It's going to be a collection of the foods you eat and their Calorie value. It may sound a "Hard task" to write down foods and Calorie values, but trust me, it isn't. If you had to write down everything available in the supermarket, then that would be a challenge!

This is no challenge, because you only have to write down the foods that you eat. Keep it Honest and Keep it Real. There are four blank pages, one for: Breakfast, Lunch, Dinner, Snacks & Beverages

You can find some pre-filled "**Quick Start**" Calorie Library Pages on my website. The items featured are some of the most common used items found in the average shopping trolly - The Calories Values are broken down into Calories Per Gram.

Your blank Calorie library pages will take you an hour or two to fill in, but trust me, it is well worth the effort and will make filling in your Diary Page really easy - **And Fast!**

Constantly update your **Calorie Library** every time you have something new. Some items vary in **Weight**, so break them down into single Calorie units.   Other items, like bread slices, eggs, sausages and so on are pretty standard so write them down as whole values. - **Portion - Serving Or Weight**

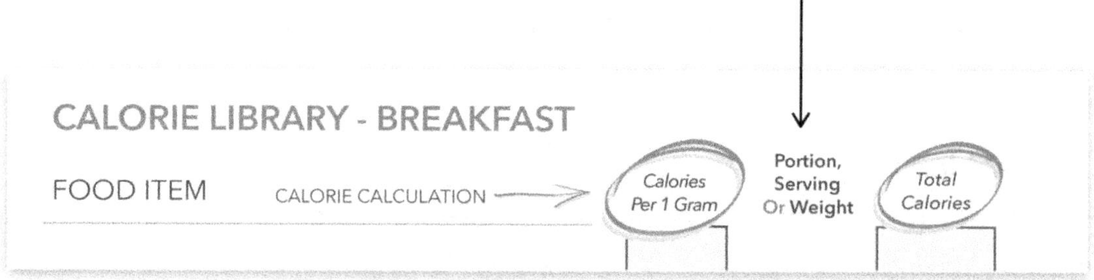

* Standard Calorie Values may vary with different brands - **Check the Packet!**
Example - Bread Slices may vary as much as 69 Calories per slice to 116 Calories per slice.

Why anything is calculated at **"Per 100 Grams"** is a complete mystery me! It's far easier to make any calculation correctly when you simply have to **"Multiply"** it.
When Breaking down "**Weight**" items into their single Calorie units, use my online **Calories Per Gram Calculator** to make life easier!   See page 32.

Required items for your success!

When you build your **Calorie Library**, use measuring spoons, measuring jug and scales.
Then once you have the calculation written down in front of you. It's so easy to refer to it.

- Measuring Spoons

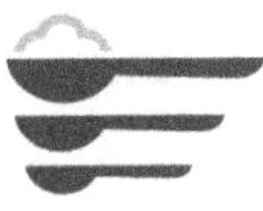

- Measuring Jug & Cups

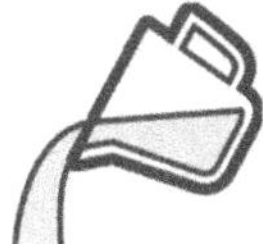

- Digital Scales

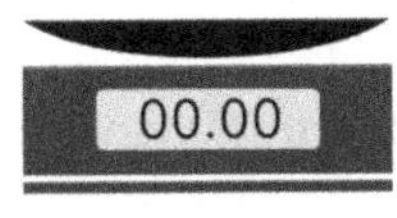

When you have built your own Calorie Library with the foods you eat, it's so easy to refer
to. Using the Calorie Library you have created - You would now know - The Calorie
content for your favourite Bread, Cheese, Pasta Sauce, Ham Slices and so on.

Where possible, when preparing your meals, use a measuring cup & spoons as you did
when you created your library. This ensures your Calorie value is near as spot on as you
can get it - **See online Videos for time saving preparation tips.**

WHEN NOT TO BOTHER!

If you are not going to eat an entire cucumber or lettuce in one sitting, then don't
bother trying to workout the Calorie values. Do add things like Tomatoes and Peppers
to your library for when you have a whole one or two in your salad.

When making a sandwich however, it's the bread, butter, meat or cheese and
condiments you want to know. Don't worry about a sprinkle of lettuce or a slice of
tomato!   Use your own judgement when it comes to super low Calorie items.

Remember to create your Beverages Library. The Calorie values for
your favourite coffee shop beverages can be found on their websites.

Remember to include all Beverages, hot and cold. And defiantly don't
forget your glass of Wine!

YOUR SET MENUS

What is a Set Menu?

A Set menu is a collection of foods from your Calorie Library all bundled together for one setting.

Breakfast example:

1 x Boiled egg	**78** Calories
1 x Slice of wholemeal bread	**51** Calories
1 x 5g (spoon of butter)	**37** Calories
1 x Bowl of porridge	**35** Calories
1 x Spoon of sugar	**16** Calories

Calorie Value for Breakfast **No.1**   **217 Calories**

Why have Set Menus?

Having a Set Menu will allow you to quickly calculate a pre-planned day's worth of Calories. Some days you may want, or need more Calories and other days less. With your Set Menus, it's very easy to do this:

☑ *For Breakfast I will have Set Menu* **No.1** *Calorie Value* **217**
☑ *For Lunch I will have Set Menu*   **No.4** *Calorie Value* **401**
☑ *For Dinner I will have Set Menu*   **No.6** *Calorie Value* **665**

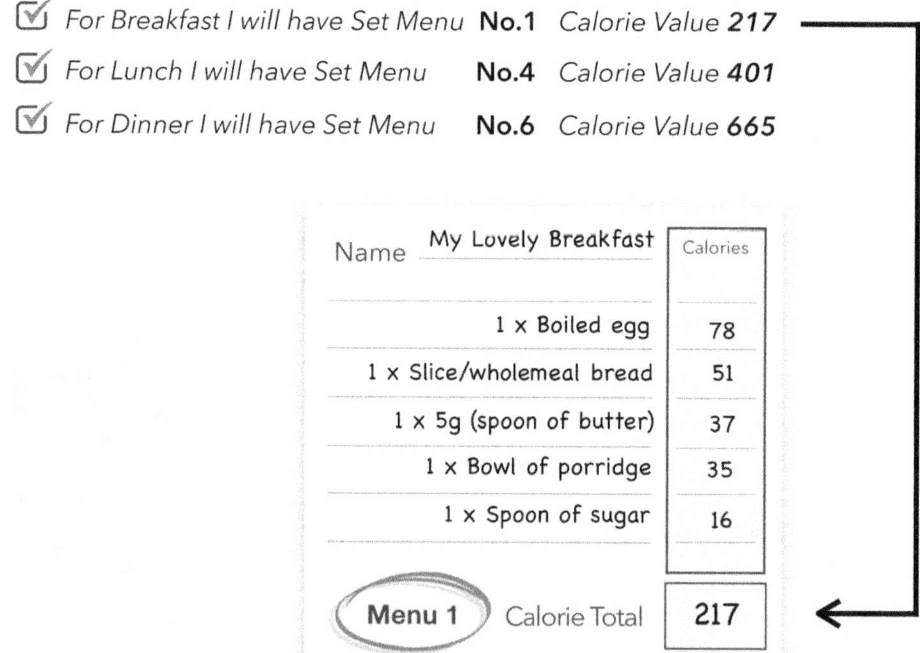

You don't have to use your set menus all the time. They are there to make your life easy, simply for those days when you are just to busy to think about meals, and Calorie calculation is far from your mind.   Sometimes your set menus will simply take away the hassle of it.

I suggest you build your menus in calorie value order, from the lowest to the highest, ranging between 200 Calories to 700 plus Calories. Having your meals vary in such Calorie values will allow you to plan your days more easily. If you have a low Calorie morning and afternoon, you can select a larger value evening meal.

Give your meal a name and total Calorie value. When recording to your Journal page, simply transfer the name and the Calorie value to the Calorie column.

Example: My Lovely Breakfast.

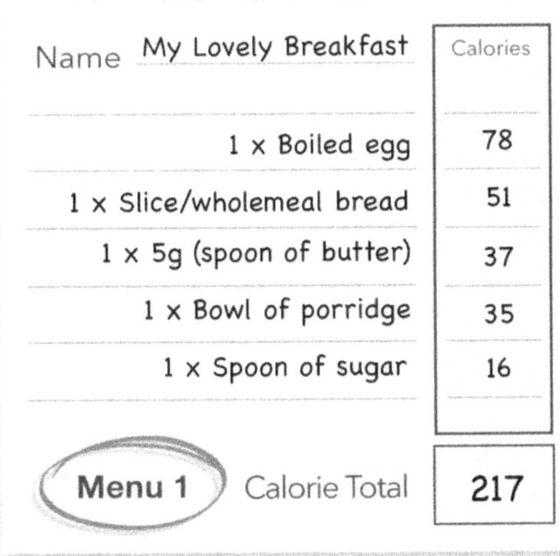

Name My Lovely Breakfast	Calories
1 x Boiled egg	78
1 x Slice/wholemeal bread	51
1 x 5g (spoon of butter)	37
1 x Bowl of porridge	35
1 x Spoon of sugar	16
(Menu 1) Calorie Total	217

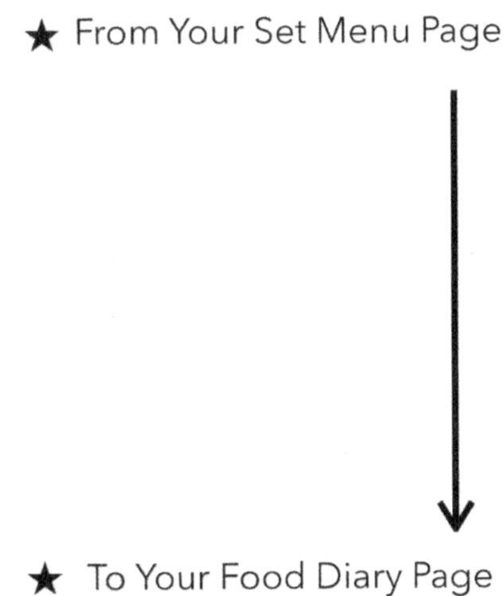

★ From Your Set Menu Page

★ To Your Food Diary Page

BREAKFAST / MORNING	Calories	✓
My Lovely Breakfast	217	

There are 38 Set Menus in total, 6 for Breakfast, 12 each for Lunch and Dinner and 8 for Snacks. If you want to build more, use a blank sheet of paper and attach it to your Diary.

SHOPPING

These dedicated sections will enable you to be more organised, which in turn will aid you in losing weight. Giving you a clear idea of what is in your food cupboard, and which day suits you best to be eating certain meals, really will benefit you.

When doing the shopping you have the necessary ingredients already outlined that you will require, whether you cook for yourself or a family. I dare say that there is even a money saving element to this in that you will no longer require to purchase those items that are not really needed. Those items like **"Buy one get one free"** and in all honesty, you had no intention of buying prior to entering the store!

SHOPPING LIST - CURRENT AND NEW (WHEN YOU ARE READY)

ITEM	CALORIE VALUE →	LOW	MED	HIGH	WHEN I'M READY SWAP FOR:

When you are ready to make some shopping basket changes - Simply look at your Higher Calorie Value Food Items and see what alternatives are available.

** Full Fat Milk for Skimmed*
** Lower Calorie Yoghurts*

and so on…

Don't do this all in one go! Take your time and change one or two items each week.

** Use a pencil, rub out and repeat with next weeks new and improved shopping list.*

AND MEAL PLANNING   *Tomorrows Meals Organised…*

When you are ready to create your Meal Planner, either a few days in advance or simply for the next day, you can use your Set Menus or simply choose something that is quick and simple.

Your Daily Food Tracking Page will also act as your Meal Planner. 

PLANNED / ACTUAL

★ When Meal Planning always use a pencil and write lightly on the page… This allows you to change your mind, rub it out and start again!

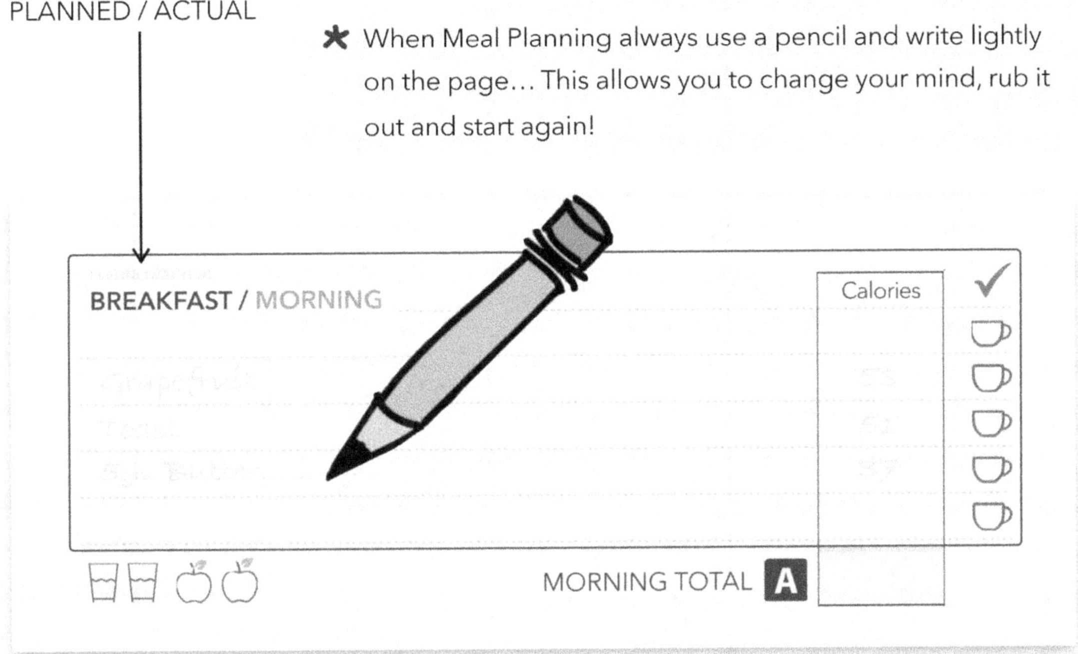

Your Meal Planner will work super well for you if you have forthcoming engagements or meals out for example. You can plan the morning and lunch time meals to be lower in Calories, allowing you more for the evening. It is simple little tips and tricks like this that will keep you organised and staying within your daily Calorie allowance.

You don't want to be to super enthusiastic at the start, there is no need to fill up all your Meal Planner section with super low, celery crunching meals from the off! This will not work, and is not honest eating. Your body requires Calories so don't set your body against you.

Only fill your Planner up a few days at a time or one week maximum and slowly make the changes when you are ready too. This allows you to make changes easily, it gives you time to get into the swing of things! Take time and think carefully about your Meal Planning!

YOUR DIARY PAGES EXPLAINED

Your **Food Diary page** has been cleverly worked out and designed to make recording your foods, beverages and calculations super easy. Everything you need is on one organised page. See the markers below and opposite page for full instructions on each feature - Simply get the best out of your day!

- 3 Calorie Sections A, B, C
- 3 Sections: Breakfast, Lunch & Dinner
- Ticks & Beverages

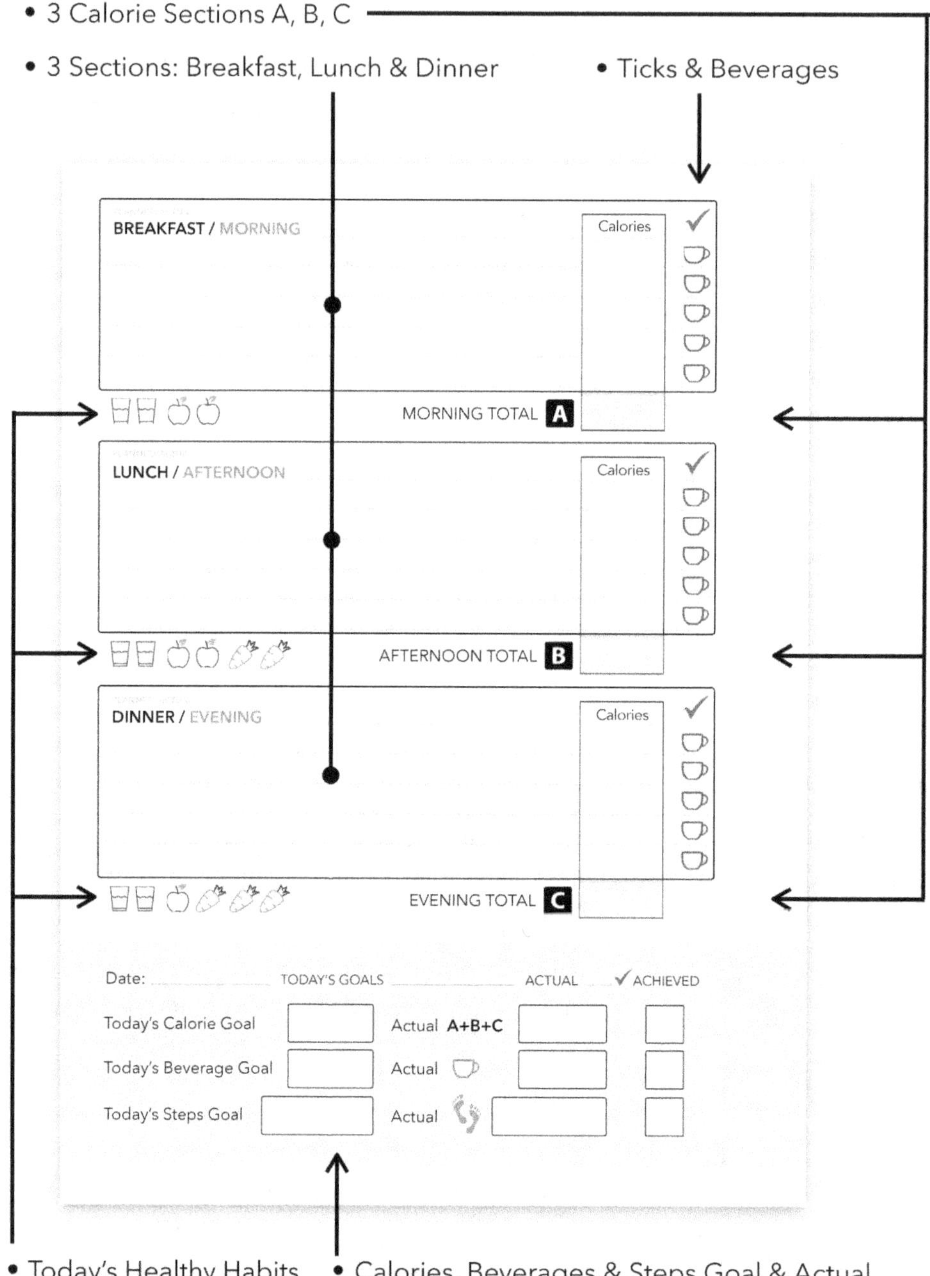

- Today's Healthy Habits
- Calories, Beverages & Steps Goal & Actual

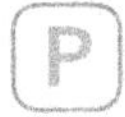 Todays Healthy Habits

There are 20 Ticks in total …
Your Daily Goal should be at least 14 to16 Ticks…

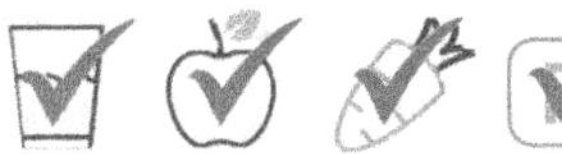

[P]   = Protein. Protein can reduce appetite, increase the feelings of fullness, decrease calorie intake and increase metabolic rate. Make sure you get plenty of it!

3 Calorie Sections - Totals A, B, C

Why are there three Calorie sections, one for Breakfast & Morning, Lunch & Afternoon and one for Dinner and Evening? There is good reason for this - This super little feature is one of the major keys to your weight loss success.

Ticks & Beverages

Ticks and Beverages. Place a tick in the beverage column each and every time you have a drink of Tea, Coffee or anything that contains Calories. (*Use your Beverage Calorie Library*)

Beverages + Sugar equal even more Calories and sometimes we drink because of habit and not hydration. Reduce your sugar over time with the Goals and Actual box. For information on how to reduce your sugar without noticing it, go to my website and select **MORE >**

Steps

Steps are a great way to burn extra calories. Have a goal and try to hit it everyday! Using a sports watch is a great way to keep you on track and also allows you to track Floors.

- Stair walking is even better at burning Calories. See online extra content for more information - Select **MORE >**

Your Daily Calorie Goal

One of the most important boxes on the page. Your Daily Calorie Allowance or Goal and your Actual Calories! You decide on a slow or how quick - You are in control. See online extra content for more information - Select **MORE >**

WHY THREE CALORIE SECTIONS?

Having three Calorie sections will make your life really easy and organised. Three Calorie sections allow you to see at a glance your Calorie totals for each section of the day, Morning, Afternoon & Evening. This information allows you to perform some handy Calorie Juggling Calculations.

Use the information to juggle and alter your Calorie intake. Because you know your Daily Calorie Goal and the Diary page is divided into three sections, you can really juggle around with your day's eating and **snacks** - Especially if you haven't had time to complete your meal planner the previous day.

A **failure point** for most Diets is going hungry when you don't have too!

At a glance, seeing your Calories in sections will help you work things out very quickly.

It's nearly the end of the day and you feel a little peckish - **Can you have that little extra?**

The answer is on your Diary Page! If you look at your Dairy Page and quickly add up your Calories **A + B + C**, then you can see if you are allowed that little extra.   Sometimes you can have as much as 300 Calories spare… That's a good treat!

Tracking your Calories this way also allows you to plan nights out or "Meal Treats"

For example: Friday night is Movie Night and you want your Binge Food - Takeaway or Delivery!

You know the Calorie Content for these "Binge Foods" because you have them in your Calorie Library - **OR SHOULD HAVE**…   Then it's a simple case of working your Calories backwards. You know what your evening Calories are going to be, so adjust your Morning and Afternoon accordingly… Simple!

For even more reasons why tracking your Calories in 3 Sections will help you succeed, please visit my website and select **MORE**.

TICKS AND BEVERAGES

Your beverages are just as important as your meals. Lots of people who are on a diet forget that beverages contain Calories. Some people drink more beverages than others. Sometimes this may be a work environment factor or simply drinking becomes a habit rather than a need.

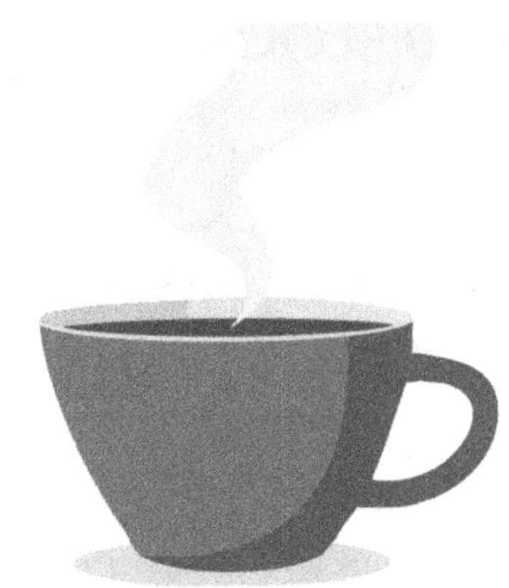

"Counting Ticks is Like Counting Calories" 

If we all took in fluids for our needs only, we would only drink water. This would be a good thing, but we don't simply drink to nourish and hydrate our bodies anymore, we drink for flavour, enjoyment and to socialise.

Beverages taste nice and supply us with a little boost or kick we are looking for. The most common beverages are, you guessed it, tea, coffee and hot chocolate.

 **+ 1 Sugar = 30 Calories x 10 Cups = 300 Calories**

The reason you need to place a tick on your Diary page each time you have a beverage, is so you can see at a glance how many beverages you are having!

You may be shocked at the amount you do have. Reducing your beverages alone may be all the difference you're looking for to lose weight.

Simply looking at the number of ticks on your page may give you a true picture to whether you are just having too many, or too many in one particular part of the day. You may be able to say to yourself - **NO** more coffees in the morning, or I will at least reduce this by half!

If you take sugar with your Tea & Coffee, we have a clever little way for you to reduce this by half, or to nothing without you even noticing it. Visit my website for more information - **> VIDEO**

STEPS AND FLOORS

There's a new personal trainer around and it comes in the form of a fitness watch. Tracking your steps is a great way to lose weight and get fit, and these clever little devices can really push you. Simply look at the watch at any point of the day and see how many steps you have taken and distance travelled.

These smart watches really do push you, and call upon your "Competitive Nature" to complete your daily goals. You will find yourself walking a lot more and constantly gauging distances against time. You will become more conscious about walking and even find yourself going the long way round, simply to add more steps to your counter.

Reports and reviews say, that some people pace the living room before going to bed so they can hit their steps goal. That's as good as having your very own personal trainer!

There are all types of watches around with varying prices ranges. To be honest you don't need an expensive one, any that track steps is all that is required and you will be able to get yourself one for less than forty pounds.

The higher the price tag the more functions you can expect to get including, seeing on your watch face who's calling you and text messages.

Walking is sometimes overlooked as a way of exercising. It's probably the easiest form of exercise there is, and will build stamina, burn calories, improve glucose levels and over time reduce your blood pressure. Experts say 10,000 steps is a good number to keep you healthy. Every step counts from around the house, office, shopping and of course "Taking a good walk". Mix it up with different routes, good music or a walking partner.

STAIR WALKING

Stair walking on the other hand is considered to be a moderate to high intensity exercise and offers even more benefits above walking. Stair walking is an amazing aerobic exercise with the added benefit of toning and strengthening your buttocks and thigh muscles. For more information about **Exercising and Weight loss**, see page 116

GETTING STARTED - SOME FOOD RULES!

☑ Food Rule No.1

Don't rush out and fill the shopping trolly up of the world's lowest Calorie food items.

Why? This is what most dieters do, and it's not sustainable. You have to take it easy and swap some food items as and when the time is ready for you to do so.

Do! Buy what you are used to, what fits in with your family and your budget! Remember your goal is to lose body fat/weight and get fit - You are not training for a marathon!

☑ Food Rule No.2

Don't set your Calorie Goal too low!

Why? Setting your Calorie Goal too low is not a long term solution. Your Body will notice a large reduction and it will not thank you! It will send signals to your brain asking for more!

Do! Play around with your Calorie Goal. Some days give yourself more and some days less. When you know your "**Daily Calorie Maintenance**" you can "Match it" or go a few hundred Calories below it. You have to train your Brain to think you're not starving!

☑ Food Rule No.3

Don't guess anything that passes your lips!

Why? The smallest of items add up. And this is where it can all go wrong big time! A single Jelly Baby Sweet contains 22 Calories - Eating just five without thinking about it is easy, but it works out to be **"110 Calories"** - Going over your daily allowance by only 130 Calories can result in a yearly weight gain of 14 pounds / 1 Stone!

Do! Track it regardless of how small or insignificant it sounds. Don't go with-out, simply track it and record it in your Diary Page. - AND YES! Even those five Jelly Babies!

SHOPPING LIST - CURRENT AND NEW *(WHEN YOU ARE READY)*

ITEM   CALORIE VALUE ⟶ | LOW | MED | HIGH | WHEN I'M READY SWAP FOR:

ITEM	CALORIE VALUE →	LOW	MED	HIGH	WHEN I'M READY SWAP FOR:
		☐	☐	☐	
		☐	☐	☐	
		☐	☐	☐	
		☐	☐	☐	
		☐	☐	☐	
		☐	☐	☐	
		☐	☐	☐	
		☐	☐	☐	
		☐	☐	☐	
		☐	☐	☐	
		☐	☐	☐	
		☐	☐	☐	
		☐	☐	☐	
		☐	☐	☐	
		☐	☐	☐	
		☐	☐	☐	
		☐	☐	☐	
		☐	☐	☐	
		☐	☐	☐	
		☐	☐	☐	
		☐	☐	☐	
		☐	☐	☐	
		☐	☐	☐	

SHOPPING LIST - CURRENT AND NEW *(WHEN YOU ARE READY)*

ITEM	CALORIE VALUE →	LOW	MED	HIGH	WHEN I'M READY SWAP FOR:

ITEM   CALORIE VALUE⟶ LOW MED HIGH   WHEN I'M READY SWAP FOR:

CALORIE LIBRARY - ONLINE CALCULATOR *Calories Per Single Gram…*

To make life easy the Calorie Value should be a single unit, then it becomes easy to work everything out.

Example: If your Ham slices are 120 Calories "**Per 100 Grams**" and your Portion weighed 50 Grams - How many Calories are in your Portion?
The Calculation would be: 120 divided by 100 x 50 = 60 Calories.

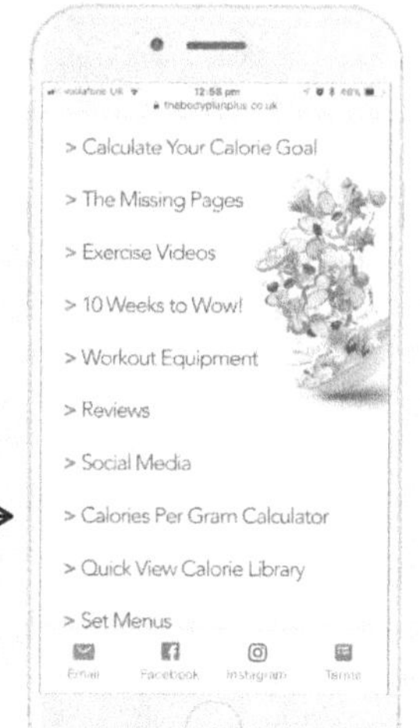

Once again you don't have to do any Calculations…. All you have to do is use my Online Calculator. Go to my website - Select **> More** and then - Calories Per Gram Calculator ⟶

VERY CLEVER!

1. Enter the Calories Per 100 Gram.

2. Enter the Portion Weight in Grams.
    Either your own Scale Weight - Or Packet Weight.

3. Hit Calculate.
    Record the information in your Calorie Library for future reference.

Calories Per Gram Calculator	
Calories (kcal) Per 100 Grams	120
Portion Weight in Grams	50
Calculate	
Calories Per Gram =	1.2
Calories in Your Portion =	60

Example: Ham

TIME SAVING TIP

When you have found the Calories Per Gram Calculator on your Mobile Device. Add the Page to your Home Screen. A small icon will appear on your phone which will allow you to open the Calculator straight away as and when you need it.

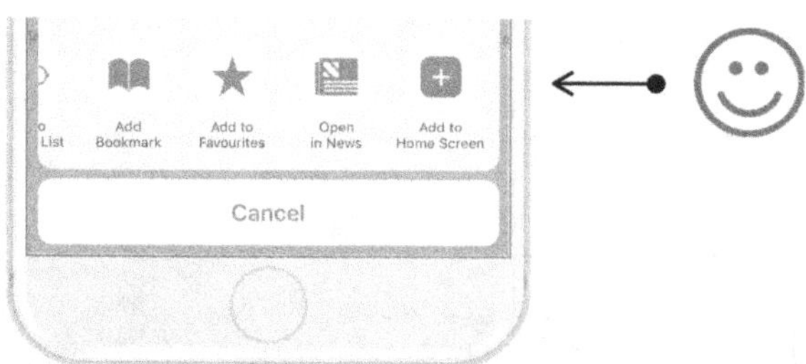

TO WORK OUT LATER...

Use this space to write down any Calculations you want to work out later!

CALORIE LIBRARY - BREAKFAST

FOOD ITEM   CALORIE CALCULATION ⟶

Calories Per 1 Gram

Portion, Serving Or Weight

Total Calories

SET MENUS *For* BREAKFAST

Name ____________________

Calories

Menu 1   Calorie Total

Name ____________________

Calories

Menu 2   Calorie Total

Name ____________________

Calories

Menu 3   Calorie Total

Name ____________________

Calories

Menu 4   Calorie Total

Name ____________________

Calories

Menu 5   Calorie Total

Name ____________________

Calories

Menu 6   Calorie Total

CALORIE LIBRARY - LUNCH

FOOD ITEM   CALORIE CALCULATION ⟶

Calories Per 1 Gram

Portion, Serving Or Weight

Total Calories

FOOD ITEM   CALORIE CALCULATION ⟶

Calories
Per 1 Gram

Portion,
Serving
Or Weight

Total
Calories

Calories
Per 1 Gram

Portion,
Serving
Or Weight

Total
Calories

SET MENUS *For* LUNCH

Name ______________________ | Calories

Menu 1   Calorie Total

Name ______________________ | Calories

Menu 4   Calorie Total

Name ______________________ | Calories

Menu 2   Calorie Total

Name ______________________ | Calories

Menu 5   Calorie Total

Name ______________________ | Calories

Menu 3   Calorie Total

Name ______________________ | Calories

Menu 6   Calorie Total

Name ___________________________

____

____

____

____

____

Calories

Menu 7 Calorie Total

Name ___________________________

____

____

____

____

____

Calories

Menu 8 Calorie Total

Name ___________________________

____

____

____

____

____

Calories

Menu 9 Calorie Total

Name ___________________________

____

____

____

____

____

Calories

Menu 10 Calorie Total

Name ___________________________

____

____

____

____

____

Calories

Menu 11 Calorie Total

Name ___________________________

____

____

____

____

____

Calories

Menu 12 Calorie Total

CALORIE LIBRARY - DINNER

FOOD ITEM   CALORIE CALCULATION ⟶

Calories Per 1 Gram

Portion, Serving Or Weight

Total Calories

FOOD ITEM

CALORIE CALCULATION ⟶

Calories Per 1 Gram

Portion, Serving Or Weight

Total Calories

SET MENUS *For* DINNER

Name ___________________________

Calories

____

____

____

____

____

Menu 1 Calorie Total

Name ___________________________

Calories

____

____

____

____

____

Menu 2 Calorie Total

Name ___________________________

Calories

____

____

____

____

____

Menu 3 Calorie Total

Name ___________________________

Calories

____

____

____

____

____

Menu 4 Calorie Total

Name ___________________________

Calories

____

____

____

____

____

Menu 5 Calorie Total

Name ___________________________

Calories

____

____

____

____

____

Menu 6 Calorie Total

Name

Calories

Menu 7 Calorie Total

Name

Calories

Menu 8 Calorie Total

Name

Calories

Menu 9 Calorie Total

Name

Calories

Menu 10 Calorie Total

Name

Calories

Menu 11 Calorie Total

Name

Calories

Menu 12 Calorie Total

CALORIE LIBRARY - SNACKS

FOOD ITEM   CALORIE CALCULATION ⟶

Calories Per 1 Gram

Portion, Serving Or Weight

Total Calories

CALORIE LIBRARY - BEVERAGES

Calories

SNACKS

FOOD ITEM   CALORIE CALCULATION ⟶

	Calories Per 1 Gram	Portion, Serving Or Weight	Total Calories

BEVERAGES

	Calories

PLANNED/ACTUAL
BREAKFAST / MORNING

Calories ✓

MORNING TOTAL **A**

PLANNED/ACTUAL
LUNCH / AFTERNOON

Calories ✓

AFTERNOON TOTAL **B**

PLANNED/ACTUAL
DINNER / EVENING

Calories ✓

EVENING TOTAL **C**

How Many Calories Can I have This Evening? **(G)** - **(A)** - **(B)** =

TODAY'S GOALS | ACTUAL | ✓ACHIEVED

Calorie Goal **G** | Actual **A+B+C** =

Beverage Goal | Actual ☕ + =

Maintenance Level | *Calories Required to Maintain Current Body Weight*

* How Many Calories Can I have This Evening? *(G)* - *(A)* - *(B)* =

TODAY'S GOALS | ACTUAL | ✓ACHIEVED

Calorie Goal **G**

Actual **A+B+C** =

Beverage Goal

Actual ⌣ + =

Maintenance Level

* Calories Required to Maintain Current Body Weight

BREAKFAST / MORNING

Calories ✓

MORNING TOTAL **A**

LUNCH / AFTERNOON

Calories ✓

AFTERNOON TOTAL **B**

DINNER / EVENING

Calories ✓

EVENING TOTAL **C**

How Many Calories Can I have This Evening? **(G)** - **(A)** - **(B)** =

	TODAY'S GOALS		ACTUAL	✓ACHIEVED
Calorie Goal **G**		Actual **A+B+C =**		
Beverage Goal		Actual ◡ + =		
Maintenance Level		*Calories Required to Maintain Current Body Weight*		

PLANNED/ACTUAL
BREAKFAST / MORNING
Calories

MORNING TOTAL **A**

PLANNED/ACTUAL
LUNCH / AFTERNOON
Calories

AFTERNOON TOTAL **B**

PLANNED/ACTUAL
DINNER / EVENING
Calories

EVENING TOTAL **C**

* *How Many Calories Can I have This Evening?* **(G)** - **(A)** - **(B)** =

TODAY'S GOALS
ACTUAL
✓ACHIEVED

Calorie Goal **G**
Actual **A+B+C** =

Beverage Goal
Actual + =

Maintenance Level
* *Calories Required to Maintain Current Body Weight*

* How Many Calories Can I have This Evening? $(G) - (A) - (B) =$

TODAY'S GOALS   ACTUAL   ✓ACHIEVED

Calorie Goal **G**   Actual **A+B+C =**

Beverage Goal   Actual ☕ **+ =**

Maintenance Level   * Calories Required to Maintain Current Body Weight

How Many Calories Can I have This Evening? **(G) - (A) - (B) =**

TODAY'S GOALS   ACTUAL ✓ACHIEVED

Calorie Goal **G**   Actual **A+B+C =**

Beverage Goal   Actual ⊃ **+ =**

Maintenance Level   *Calories Required to Maintain Current Body Weight*

BREAKFAST / MORNING

Calories ✓

MORNING TOTAL **A**

LUNCH / AFTERNOON

Calories ✓

AFTERNOON TOTAL **B**

DINNER / EVENING

Calories ✓

EVENING TOTAL **C**

*How Many Calories Can I have This Evening? **(G) - (A) - (B) =***

	TODAY'S GOALS		ACTUAL	✓ACHIEVED
Calorie Goal **G**		Actual **A+B+C =**		
Beverage Goal		Actual ⎕ **+ =**		
Maintenance Level		*Calories Required to Maintain Current Body Weight*		

BREAKFAST / MORNING

Calories

✓

MORNING TOTAL **A**

LUNCH / AFTERNOON

Calories

✓

AFTERNOON TOTAL **B**

DINNER / EVENING

Calories

✓

EVENING TOTAL **C**

How Many Calories Can I have This Evening? **(G) - (A) - (B) =**

TODAY'S GOALS | ACTUAL | ✓ACHIEVED

Calorie Goal **G**

Actual **A+B+C =**

Beverage Goal

Actual ☕ **+ =**

Maintenance Level

Calories Required to Maintain Current Body Weight

BREAKFAST / MORNING

Calories

MORNING TOTAL **A**

LUNCH / AFTERNOON

Calories

AFTERNOON TOTAL **B**

DINNER / EVENING

Calories

EVENING TOTAL **C**

How Many Calories Can I have This Evening? **(G) - (A) - (B) =**

TODAY'S GOALS   ACTUAL   ✓ACHIEVED

Calorie Goal **G**   Actual **A+B+C =**

Beverage Goal   Actual ☕ + =

Maintenance Level   *Calories Required to Maintain Current Body Weight*

How Many Calories Can I have This Evening? **(G) - (A) - (B) =**

TODAY'S GOALS   ACTUAL   ✓ACHIEVED

Calorie Goal **G**

Actual **A+B+C =**

Beverage Goal

Actual + =

Maintenance Level

* *Calories Required to Maintain Current Body Weight*

* How Many Calories Can I have This Evening? *(G) - (A) - (B) =*

	TODAY'S GOALS		ACTUAL	✓ACHIEVED
Calorie Goal **G**		Actual **A+B+C =**		
Beverage Goal		Actual ☕ + =		
Maintenance Level		* Calories Required to Maintain Current Body Weight		

BREAKFAST / MORNING

Calories

MORNING TOTAL **A**

LUNCH / AFTERNOON

Calories

AFTERNOON TOTAL **B**

DINNER / EVENING

Calories

EVENING TOTAL **C**

How Many Calories Can I have This Evening? **(G)** - **(A)** - **(B)** =

	TODAY'S GOALS		ACTUAL	✓ ACHIEVED
Calorie Goal **G**		Actual **A+B+C** =		
Beverage Goal		Actual ☕ + =		
Maintenance Level		*Calories Required to Maintain Current Body Weight*		

BREAKFAST / MORNING

Calories

MORNING TOTAL **A**

LUNCH / AFTERNOON

Calories

AFTERNOON TOTAL **B**

DINNER / EVENING

Calories

EVENING TOTAL **C**

* How Many Calories Can I have This Evening? **(G)** - **(A)** - **(B)** =

TODAY'S GOALS | ACTUAL | ✓ACHIEVED

Calorie Goal **G**

Actual **A+B+C** =

Beverage Goal

Actual + =

Maintenance Level

* Calories Required to Maintain Current Body Weight

* How Many Calories Can I have This Evening? **(G)** - **(A)** - **(B)** =

TODAY'S GOALS   ACTUAL   ✓ACHIEVED

Calorie Goal **G**   Actual **A+B+C** =

Beverage Goal   Actual ☕ + =

Maintenance Level   * Calories Required to Maintain Current Body Weight

BREAKFAST / MORNING

Calories

MORNING TOTAL **A**

LUNCH / AFTERNOON

Calories

AFTERNOON TOTAL **B**

DINNER / EVENING

Calories

EVENING TOTAL **C**

How Many Calories Can I have This Evening? **(G) - (A) - (B) =**

TODAY'S GOALS

ACTUAL ✓ACHIEVED

Calorie Goal **G**

Actual **A+B+C =**

Beverage Goal

Actual ⌣ **+ =**

Maintenance Level

Calories Required to Maintain Current Body Weight

How Many Calories Can I have This Evening? **(G)** - **(A)** - **(B)** =

TODAY'S GOALS   ACTUAL ✓ACHIEVED

Calorie Goal **G**   Actual **A+B+C =**

Beverage Goal   Actual ☕ + =

Maintenance Level   *Calories Required to Maintain Current Body Weight*

How Many Calories Can I have This Evening? **(G) - (A) - (B) =**

TODAY'S GOALS   ACTUAL   ✓ACHIEVED

Calorie Goal **G**   Actual **A+B+C =**

Beverage Goal   Actual ☕ **+ =**

Maintenance Level   *Calories Required to Maintain Current Body Weight*

BREAKFAST / MORNING

Calories

MORNING TOTAL **A**

LUNCH / AFTERNOON

Calories

AFTERNOON TOTAL **B**

DINNER / EVENING

Calories

EVENING TOTAL **C**

** How Many Calories Can I have This Evening?* **(G) - (A) - (B) =**

TODAY'S GOALS

ACTUAL ✓ACHIEVED

Calorie Goal **G**

Actual **A+B+C =**

Beverage Goal

Actual ☕ **+ =**

Maintenance Level

** Calories Required to Maintain Current Body Weight*

PLANNED/ACTUAL
BREAKFAST / MORNING

Calories ✓

MORNING TOTAL **A**

PLANNED/ACTUAL
LUNCH / AFTERNOON

Calories ✓

AFTERNOON TOTAL **B**

PLANNED/ACTUAL
DINNER / EVENING

Calories ✓

EVENING TOTAL **C**

How Many Calories Can I have This Evening? **(G)** - **(A)** - **(B)** =

TODAY'S GOALS   ACTUAL   ✓ACHIEVED

Calorie Goal **G**   Actual **A+B+C** =

Beverage Goal   Actual ☕ **+** =

Maintenance Level   *Calories Required to Maintain Current Body Weight*

BREAKFAST / MORNING

Calories

MORNING TOTAL **A**

LUNCH / AFTERNOON

Calories

AFTERNOON TOTAL **B**

DINNER / EVENING

Calories

EVENING TOTAL **C**

How Many Calories Can I have This Evening? **(G) - (A) - (B)** =

	TODAY'S GOALS		ACTUAL	✓ACHIEVED
Calorie Goal **G**		Actual **A+B+C** =		
Beverage Goal		Actual ☕ + =		
Maintenance Level		*Calories Required to Maintain Current Body Weight*		

How Many Calories Can I have This Evening? (G) - (A) - (B) =

	TODAY'S GOALS		ACTUAL	✓ACHIEVED
Calorie Goal G		Actual A+B+C =		
Beverage Goal		Actual ☕ + =		
Maintenance Level		*Calories Required to Maintain Current Body Weight*		

* *How Many Calories Can I have This Evening?* **(G) - (A) - (B) =**

TODAY'S GOALS   ACTUAL   ✓ACHIEVED

Calorie Goal **G**

Actual **A+B+C =**

Beverage Goal

Actual ⌣ **+ =**

Maintenance Level

* *Calories Required to Maintain Current Body Weight*

How Many Calories Can I have This Evening? **(G) - (A) - (B) =**

	TODAY'S GOALS		ACTUAL	✓ACHIEVED
Calorie Goal **G**		Actual **A+B+C =**		
Beverage Goal		Actual ☕ **+ =**		
Maintenance Level				

Calories Required to Maintain Current Body Weight

* How Many Calories Can I have This Evening? (G) - (A) - (B) =

TODAY'S GOALS   ACTUAL   ✓ACHIEVED

Calorie Goal G

Actual A+B+C =

Beverage Goal

Actual ⌣ + =

Maintenance Level

* Calories Required to Maintain Current Body Weight

BREAKFAST / MORNING

Calories

MORNING TOTAL **A**

LUNCH / AFTERNOON

Calories

AFTERNOON TOTAL **B**

DINNER / EVENING

Calories

EVENING TOTAL **C**

How Many Calories Can I have This Evening? **(G) - (A) - (B) =**

TODAY'S GOALS   ACTUAL   ✓ACHIEVED

Calorie Goal **G**

Actual **A+B+C =**

Beverage Goal

Actual ☕ **+ =**

Maintenance Level

Calories Required to Maintain Current Body Weight

BREAKFAST / MORNING

Calories ✓

MORNING TOTAL **A**

LUNCH / AFTERNOON

Calories ✓

AFTERNOON TOTAL **B**

DINNER / EVENING

Calories ✓

EVENING TOTAL **C**

** How Many Calories Can I have This Evening?* **(G) - (A) - (B) =**

TODAY'S GOALS   ACTUAL   ✓ACHIEVED

Calorie Goal **G**

Actual **A+B+C =**

Beverage Goal

Actual 🍵 **+ =**

Maintenance Level

** Calories Required to Maintain Current Body Weight*

PLANNED/ACTUAL

BREAKFAST / MORNING

Calories ✓

MORNING TOTAL **A**

PLANNED/ACTUAL

LUNCH / AFTERNOON

Calories ✓

AFTERNOON TOTAL **B**

PLANNED/ACTUAL

DINNER / EVENING

Calories ✓

EVENING TOTAL **C**

** How Many Calories Can I have This Evening?* **(G) - (A) - (B) =**

TODAY'S GOALS | ACTUAL | ✓ACHIEVED

Calorie Goal **G** | Actual **A+B+C =**

Beverage Goal | Actual ⌣ **+ =**

Maintenance Level | ** Calories Required to Maintain Current Body Weight*

BREAKFAST / MORNING

Calories

MORNING TOTAL **A**

LUNCH / AFTERNOON

Calories

AFTERNOON TOTAL **B**

DINNER / EVENING

Calories

EVENING TOTAL **C**

* How Many Calories Can I have This Evening? **(G)** - **(A)** - **(B)** =

TODAY'S GOALS   ACTUAL   ✓ACHIEVED

Calorie Goal **G**

Actual **A+B+C** =

Beverage Goal

Actual ☕ + =

Maintenance Level

* Calories Required to Maintain Current Body Weight

BREAKFAST / MORNING

Calories

MORNING TOTAL **A**

LUNCH / AFTERNOON

Calories

AFTERNOON TOTAL **B**

DINNER / EVENING

Calories

EVENING TOTAL **C**

** How Many Calories Can I have This Evening?* **(G) - (A) - (B) =**

TODAY'S GOALS   ACTUAL   ✓ACHIEVED

Calorie Goal **G**

Actual **A+B+C =**

Beverage Goal

Actual ☕ + =

Maintenance Level

** Calories Required to Maintain Current Body Weight*

BREAKFAST / MORNING

Calories

MORNING TOTAL **A**

LUNCH / AFTERNOON

Calories

AFTERNOON TOTAL **B**

DINNER / EVENING

Calories

EVENING TOTAL **C**

* How Many Calories Can I have This Evening? **(G) - (A) - (B) =**

TODAY'S GOALS   ACTUAL   ✓ACHIEVED

Calorie Goal **G**

Actual **A+B+C =**

Beverage Goal

Actual ☕ **+ =**

Maintenance Level

* Calories Required to Maintain Current Body Weight

BREAKFAST / MORNING

Calories

MORNING TOTAL **A**

LUNCH / AFTERNOON

Calories

AFTERNOON TOTAL **B**

DINNER / EVENING

Calories

EVENING TOTAL **C**

** How Many Calories Can I have This Evening?* **(G) - (A) - (B) =**

TODAY'S GOALS | ACTUAL | ✓ACHIEVED

Calorie Goal **G**

Actual **A+B+C =**

Beverage Goal

Actual ☕ **+ =**

Maintenance Level

** Calories Required to Maintain Current Body Weight*

PLANNED/ACTUAL
BREAKFAST / MORNING
Calories
MORNING TOTAL A

PLANNED/ACTUAL
LUNCH / AFTERNOON
Calories
AFTERNOON TOTAL B

PLANNED/ACTUAL
DINNER / EVENING
Calories
EVENING TOTAL C

* How Many Calories Can I have This Evening? (G) - (A) - (B) =

TODAY'S GOALS
ACTUAL
✓ACHIEVED
Calorie Goal G
Actual A+B+C =
Beverage Goal
Actual ☕ + =
Maintenance Level
* Calories Required to Maintain Current Body Weight

BREAKFAST / MORNING

Calories

MORNING TOTAL **A**

LUNCH / AFTERNOON

Calories

AFTERNOON TOTAL **B**

DINNER / EVENING

Calories

EVENING TOTAL **C**

* *How Many Calories Can I have This Evening?* **(G) - (A) - (B)** =

TODAY'S GOALS   ACTUAL   ✓ACHIEVED

Calorie Goal **G**   Actual **A+B+C** =

Beverage Goal   Actual 🍵 + =

Maintenance Level   * *Calories Required to Maintain Current Body Weight*

PLANNED/ACTUAL
BREAKFAST / MORNING
Calories
MORNING TOTAL A

PLANNED/ACTUAL
LUNCH / AFTERNOON
Calories
AFTERNOON TOTAL B

PLANNED/ACTUAL
DINNER / EVENING
Calories
EVENING TOTAL C

* How Many Calories Can I have This Evening? (G) - (A) - (B) =

TODAY'S GOALS
ACTUAL
✓ACHIEVED

Calorie Goal G
Actual A+B+C =

Beverage Goal
Actual + =

Maintenance Level
* Calories Required to Maintain Current Body Weight

BREAKFAST / MORNING

Calories

MORNING TOTAL **A**

LUNCH / AFTERNOON

Calories

AFTERNOON TOTAL **B**

DINNER / EVENING

Calories

EVENING TOTAL **C**

*How Many Calories Can I have This Evening? (**G**) - (**A**) - (**B**) =*

TODAY'S GOALS ACTUAL ✓ACHIEVED

Calorie Goal **G** Actual **A+B+C =**

Beverage Goal Actual ⌣ **+ =**

Maintenance Level *Calories Required to Maintain Current Body Weight*

BREAKFAST / MORNING

Calories

MORNING TOTAL **A**

LUNCH / AFTERNOON

Calories

AFTERNOON TOTAL **B**

DINNER / EVENING

Calories

EVENING TOTAL **C**

* How Many Calories Can I have This Evening? **(G)** - **(A)** - **(B)** =

	TODAY'S GOALS		ACTUAL	✓ACHIEVED
Calorie Goal **G**		Actual **A+B+C** =		
Beverage Goal		Actual ☕ + =		
Maintenance Level		* Calories Required to Maintain Current Body Weight		

* *How Many Calories Can I have This Evening?* **(G) - (A) - (B) =**

	TODAY'S GOALS		ACTUAL	✓ ACHIEVED
Calorie Goal **G**		Actual **A+B+C =**		
Beverage Goal		Actual ☕ **+ =**		
Maintenance Level		*Calories Required to Maintain Current Body Weight*		

BREAKFAST / MORNING

Calories

MORNING TOTAL **A**

LUNCH / AFTERNOON

Calories

AFTERNOON TOTAL **B**

DINNER / EVENING

Calories

EVENING TOTAL **C**

* *How Many Calories Can I have This Evening?* **(G)** - **(A)** - **(B)** =

TODAY'S GOALS   ACTUAL   ✓ACHIEVED

Calorie Goal **G**   Actual **A+B+C** =

Beverage Goal   Actual ☕ **+** =

Maintenance Level   ** Calories Required to Maintain Current Body Weight*

* How Many Calories Can I have This Evening? **(G) - (A) - (B) =**

	TODAY'S GOALS		ACTUAL	✓ACHIEVED
Calorie Goal **G**		Actual **A+B+C =**		
Beverage Goal		Actual ☕ **+ =**		
Maintenance Level		* Calories Required to Maintain Current Body Weight		

BREAKFAST / MORNING

Calories

MORNING TOTAL **A**

LUNCH / AFTERNOON

Calories

AFTERNOON TOTAL **B**

DINNER / EVENING

Calories

EVENING TOTAL **C**

How Many Calories Can I have This Evening? (G) - (A) - (B) =

TODAY'S GOALS | ACTUAL | ✓ACHIEVED

Calorie Goal **G**

Actual **A+B+C =**

Beverage Goal

Actual + =

Maintenance Level

Calories Required to Maintain Current Body Weight

BREAKFAST / MORNING

Calories

MORNING TOTAL **A**

LUNCH / AFTERNOON

Calories

AFTERNOON TOTAL **B**

DINNER / EVENING

Calories

EVENING TOTAL **C**

** How Many Calories Can I have This Evening?* **(G) - (A) - (B) =**

TODAY'S GOALS   ACTUAL   ✓ACHIEVED

Calorie Goal **G**   Actual **A+B+C =**

Beverage Goal   Actual ☕ **+ =**

Maintenance Level   ** Calories Required to Maintain Current Body Weight*

PLANNED/ACTUAL
BREAKFAST / MORNING

Calories ✓

MORNING TOTAL **A**

PLANNED/ACTUAL
LUNCH / AFTERNOON

Calories ✓

AFTERNOON TOTAL **B**

PLANNED/ACTUAL
DINNER / EVENING

Calories ✓

EVENING TOTAL **C**

How Many Calories Can I have This Evening? **(G) - (A) - (B) =**

TODAY'S GOALS   ACTUAL   ✓ACHIEVED

Calorie Goal **G**

Actual **A+B+C =**

Beverage Goal

Actual ☕ **+ =**

Maintenance Level

Calories Required to Maintain Current Body Weight

BREAKFAST / MORNING

Calories

MORNING TOTAL **A**

LUNCH / AFTERNOON

Calories

AFTERNOON TOTAL **B**

DINNER / EVENING

Calories

EVENING TOTAL **C**

How Many Calories Can I have This Evening? **(G) - (A) - (B) =**

TODAY'S GOALS   ACTUAL   ✓ACHIEVED

Calorie Goal **G**   Actual **A+B+C =**

Beverage Goal   Actual ☕ **+ =**

Maintenance Level   *Calories Required to Maintain Current Body Weight*

PLANNED/ACTUAL
BREAKFAST / MORNING
Calories
MORNING TOTAL A

PLANNED/ACTUAL
LUNCH / AFTERNOON
Calories
AFTERNOON TOTAL B

PLANNED/ACTUAL
DINNER / EVENING
Calories
EVENING TOTAL C

* How Many Calories Can I have This Evening? (G) - (A) - (B) =

TODAY'S GOALS   ACTUAL   ✓ACHIEVED
Calorie Goal G   Actual A+B+C =
Beverage Goal   Actual ⌣ + =
Maintenance Level   * Calories Required to Maintain Current Body Weight

PLANNED/ACTUAL
BREAKFAST / MORNING
Calories
MORNING TOTAL A

PLANNED/ACTUAL
LUNCH / AFTERNOON
Calories
AFTERNOON TOTAL B

PLANNED/ACTUAL
DINNER / EVENING
Calories
EVENING TOTAL C

* How Many Calories Can I have This Evening? (G) - (A) - (B) =

TODAY'S GOALS   ACTUAL   ✓ACHIEVED

Calorie Goal G   Actual A+B+C =

Beverage Goal   Actual   + =

Maintenance Level   * Calories Required to Maintain Current Body Weight

How Many Calories Can I have This Evening? (G) - (A) - (B) =

	TODAY'S GOALS		ACTUAL	✓ACHIEVED
Calorie Goal **G**		Actual **A+B+C =**		
Beverage Goal		Actual ☕ **+** **=**		
Maintenance Level		*Calories Required to Maintain Current Body Weight*		

BREAKFAST / MORNING

Calories

MORNING TOTAL **A**

LUNCH / AFTERNOON

Calories

AFTERNOON TOTAL **B**

DINNER / EVENING

Calories

EVENING TOTAL **C**

How Many Calories Can I have This Evening? **(G) - (A) - (B) =**

TODAY'S GOALS | ACTUAL | ✓ACHIEVED

Calorie Goal **G**

Actual **A+B+C =**

Beverage Goal

Actual + =

Maintenance Level

Calories Required to Maintain Current Body Weight

PLANNED/ACTUAL
BREAKFAST / MORNING
Calories
MORNING TOTAL A

PLANNED/ACTUAL
LUNCH / AFTERNOON
Calories
AFTERNOON TOTAL B

PLANNED/ACTUAL
DINNER / EVENING
Calories
EVENING TOTAL C

* How Many Calories Can I have This Evening? (G) - (A) - (B) =

TODAY'S GOALS   ACTUAL   ✓ACHIEVED
Calorie Goal G   Actual A+B+C =
Beverage Goal   Actual ☕ + =
Maintenance Level   * Calories Required to Maintain Current Body Weight

PLANNED/ACTUAL
BREAKFAST / MORNING

Calories ✓

MORNING TOTAL **A**

PLANNED/ACTUAL
LUNCH / AFTERNOON

Calories ✓

AFTERNOON TOTAL **B**

PLANNED/ACTUAL
DINNER / EVENING

Calories ✓

EVENING TOTAL **C**

** How Many Calories Can I have This Evening?* **(G) - (A) - (B) =**

TODAY'S GOALS   ACTUAL   ✓ACHIEVED

Calorie Goal **G**   Actual **A+B+C =**

Beverage Goal   Actual ☕ **+ =**

Maintenance Level   ** Calories Required to Maintain Current Body Weight*

*How Many Calories Can I have This Evening? **(G) - (A) - (B) =**

TODAY'S GOALS   ACTUAL   ✓ACHIEVED

Calorie Goal **G**   Actual **A+B+C =**

Beverage Goal   Actual ⬭ + =

Maintenance Level   *Calories Required to Maintain Current Body Weight*

How Many Calories Can I have This Evening? **(G) - (A) - (B) =**

TODAY'S GOALS   ACTUAL   ✓ACHIEVED

Calorie Goal **G**   Actual **A+B+C =**

Beverage Goal   Actual   + =

Maintenance Level   *Calories Required to Maintain Current Body Weight*

BREAKFAST / MORNING

Calories

MORNING TOTAL **A**

LUNCH / AFTERNOON

Calories

AFTERNOON TOTAL **B**

DINNER / EVENING

Calories

EVENING TOTAL **C**

How Many Calories Can I have This Evening? **(G)** - **(A)** - **(B)** =

TODAY'S GOALS · ACTUAL · ✓ACHIEVED

Calorie Goal **G**

Actual **A+B+C** =

Beverage Goal

Actual ☕ + =

Maintenance Level

Calories Required to Maintain Current Body Weight

*How Many Calories Can I have This Evening? **(G) - (A) - (B)** =

TODAY'S GOALS   ACTUAL   ✓ACHIEVED

Calorie Goal **G**   Actual **A+B+C** =

Beverage Goal   Actual ☕ + =

Maintenance Level   *Calories Required to Maintain Current Body Weight*

* How Many Calories Can I have This Evening? *(G)* - *(A)* - *(B)* =

	TODAY'S GOALS		ACTUAL	✓ACHIEVED
Calorie Goal **G**		Actual **A+B+C** =		
Beverage Goal		Actual ☕ + =		
Maintenance Level		* Calories Required to Maintain Current Body Weight		

* How Many Calories Can I have This Evening? **(G) - (A) - (B) =**

BREAKFAST / MORNING

Calories ✓

MORNING TOTAL **A**

LUNCH / AFTERNOON

Calories ✓

AFTERNOON TOTAL **B**

DINNER / EVENING

Calories ✓

EVENING TOTAL **C**

How Many Calories Can I have This Evening? **(G) - (A) - (B) =**

TODAY'S GOALS   ACTUAL   ✓ACHIEVED

Calorie Goal **G**

Actual **A+B+C =**

Beverage Goal

Actual ⌣ **+ =**

Maintenance Level

Calories Required to Maintain Current Body Weight

PLANNED/ACTUAL
BREAKFAST / MORNING

Calories ✓

MORNING TOTAL **A**

PLANNED/ACTUAL
LUNCH / AFTERNOON

Calories ✓

AFTERNOON TOTAL **B**

PLANNED/ACTUAL
DINNER / EVENING

Calories ✓

EVENING TOTAL **C**

*How Many Calories Can I have This Evening? **(G) - (A) - (B)** =

TODAY'S GOALS | | ACTUAL | ✓ACHIEVED

Calorie Goal **G** | | Actual **A+B+C =**

Beverage Goal | | Actual ☕ **+** =

Maintenance Level | *Calories Required to Maintain Current Body Weight*

How Many Calories Can I have This Evening? **(G) - (A) - (B) =**

TODAY'S GOALS | ACTUAL | ✓ACHIEVED

Calorie Goal **G**

Actual **A+B+C =**

Beverage Goal

Actual ☕ **+ =**

Maintenance Level

Calories Required to Maintain Current Body Weight

BREAKFAST / MORNING

Calories ✓

MORNING TOTAL **A**

LUNCH / AFTERNOON

Calories ✓

AFTERNOON TOTAL **B**

DINNER / EVENING

Calories ✓

EVENING TOTAL **C**

*How Many Calories Can I have This Evening? **(G)** - **(A)** - **(B)** =

TODAY'S GOALS · · · · · · ACTUAL · ✓ACHIEVED

Calorie Goal **G**

Actual **A+B+C =**

Beverage Goal

Actual ⌣ + =

Maintenance Level

*Calories Required to Maintain Current Body Weight

PLANNED/ACTUAL

BREAKFAST / MORNING

Calories ✓

MORNING TOTAL **A**

PLANNED/ACTUAL

LUNCH / AFTERNOON

Calories ✓

AFTERNOON TOTAL **B**

PLANNED/ACTUAL

DINNER / EVENING

Calories ✓

EVENING TOTAL **C**

How Many Calories Can I have This Evening? **(G) - (A) - (B) =**

TODAY'S GOALS   ACTUAL   ✓ACHIEVED

Calorie Goal **G**

Actual **A+B+C =**

Beverage Goal

Actual ☕ **+ =**

Maintenance Level

* Calories Required to Maintain Current Body Weight

BREAKFAST / MORNING

Calories

MORNING TOTAL **A**

LUNCH / AFTERNOON

Calories

AFTERNOON TOTAL **B**

DINNER / EVENING

Calories

EVENING TOTAL **C**

* *How Many Calories Can I have This Evening?* **(G)** - **(A)** - **(B)** =

	TODAY'S GOALS		ACTUAL	✓ACHIEVED
Calorie Goal **G**		Actual **A+B+C** =		
Beverage Goal		Actual ☕ + =		
Maintenance Level		* Calories Required to Maintain Current Body Weight		

PLANNED/ACTUAL

BREAKFAST / MORNING

Calories ✓

MORNING TOTAL **A**

PLANNED/ACTUAL

LUNCH / AFTERNOON

Calories ✓

AFTERNOON TOTAL **B**

PLANNED/ACTUAL

DINNER / EVENING

Calories ✓

EVENING TOTAL **C**

How Many Calories Can I have This Evening? **(G)** - **(A)** - **(B)** =

TODAY'S GOALS | ACTUAL | ✓ACHIEVED

Calorie Goal **G** | Actual **A+B+C** =

Beverage Goal | Actual ☕ **+** =

Maintenance Level | *Calories Required to Maintain Current Body Weight*

How Many Calories Can I have This Evening? **(G) - (A) - (B) =**

TODAY'S GOALS | ACTUAL | ✓ACHIEVED

Calorie Goal **G** | Actual **A+B+C =**

Beverage Goal | Actual ☕ + =

Maintenance Level | *Calories Required to Maintain Current Body Weight*

PLANNED/ACTUAL
BREAKFAST / MORNING
Calories
MORNING TOTAL A

PLANNED/ACTUAL
LUNCH / AFTERNOON
Calories
AFTERNOON TOTAL B

PLANNED/ACTUAL
DINNER / EVENING
Calories
EVENING TOTAL C

* How Many Calories Can I have This Evening? (G) - (A) - (B) =

TODAY'S GOALS   ACTUAL   ✓ACHIEVED
Calorie Goal G   Actual A+B+C =
Beverage Goal   Actual ☕ + =
Maintenance Level   * Calories Required to Maintain Current Body Weight

PLANNED/ACTUAL

BREAKFAST / MORNING

Calories ✓

MORNING TOTAL **A**

PLANNED/ACTUAL

LUNCH / AFTERNOON

Calories ✓

AFTERNOON TOTAL **B**

PLANNED/ACTUAL

DINNER / EVENING

Calories ✓

EVENING TOTAL **C**

** How Many Calories Can I have This Evening?* **(G)** - **(A)** - **(B)** =

TODAY'S GOALS   ACTUAL   ✓ACHIEVED

Calorie Goal **G**   Actual **A+B+C** =

Beverage Goal   Actual ☕ + =

Maintenance Level   ** Calories Required to Maintain Current Body Weight*

BREAKFAST / MORNING

Calories

MORNING TOTAL **A**

LUNCH / AFTERNOON

Calories

AFTERNOON TOTAL **B**

DINNER / EVENING

Calories

EVENING TOTAL **C**

How Many Calories Can I have This Evening? **(G)** - **(A)** - **(B)** =

TODAY'S GOALS — ACTUAL — ✓ACHIEVED

Calorie Goal **G** — Actual **A+B+C =**

Beverage Goal — Actual ☕ **+ =**

Maintenance Level — *Calories Required to Maintain Current Body Weight*

How Many Calories Can I have This Evening? **(G) - (A) - (B) =**

TODAY'S GOALS
ACTUAL
✓ACHIEVED

Calorie Goal **G**
Actual **A+B+C =**

Beverage Goal
Actual + =

Maintenance Level
Calories Required to Maintain Current Body Weight

* How Many Calories Can I have This Evening? **(G) - (A) - (B) =**

	TODAY'S GOALS		ACTUAL	✓ACHIEVED
Calorie Goal **G**		Actual **A+B+C =**		
Beverage Goal		Actual ⌣ + =		
Maintenance Level		* Calories Required to Maintain Current Body Weight		

How Many Calories Can I have This Evening? **(G) - (A) - (B) =**

TODAY'S GOALS   ACTUAL   ✓ACHIEVED

Calorie Goal **G**

Actual **A+B+C =**

Beverage Goal

Actual + =

Maintenance Level

Calories Required to Maintain Current Body Weight

BREAKFAST / MORNING

Calories ✓

MORNING TOTAL **A**

LUNCH / AFTERNOON

Calories ✓

AFTERNOON TOTAL **B**

DINNER / EVENING

Calories ✓

EVENING TOTAL **C**

How Many Calories Can I have This Evening? **(G) - (A) - (B) =**

TODAY'S GOALS | ACTUAL | ✓ACHIEVED

Calorie Goal **G**

Actual **A+B+C =**

Beverage Goal

Actual ☕ **+ =**

Maintenance Level

Calories Required to Maintain Current Body Weight

ABOUT ME AND MY MOTIVATION

☑ **ABOUT ME:** *Write down the things I like... What makes me, me?*

☑ **GOALS:** *What are my Goals... What motivates me?*

☑ **WHY:** *Write down why I want to make changes in my life!*

☑ **EXERCISE:** *What Exercises will I be doing to speed things up?*

☑ **FOCUS:** *Statement to myself, that will keep me focused!*

WEIGHT TRACKER GRAPH

Enter your "**Stone**" Weight only in **Box A** - then mark on the graph your "**Pound**" Weight!

HOW MUCH AND HOW FAST?

You are looking to lose a healthy 1 to 1 and a half pound per week. Any more than this and your body may go into starvation mode. You want to avoid this at all costs because this may result in failure To avoid this and ensure success go to my help page for more information and how to avoid this situation. "**Success is yours with a little knowledge** "

To avoid Starvation mode, visit the website and select **MORE>** and then find the "Missing Pages"

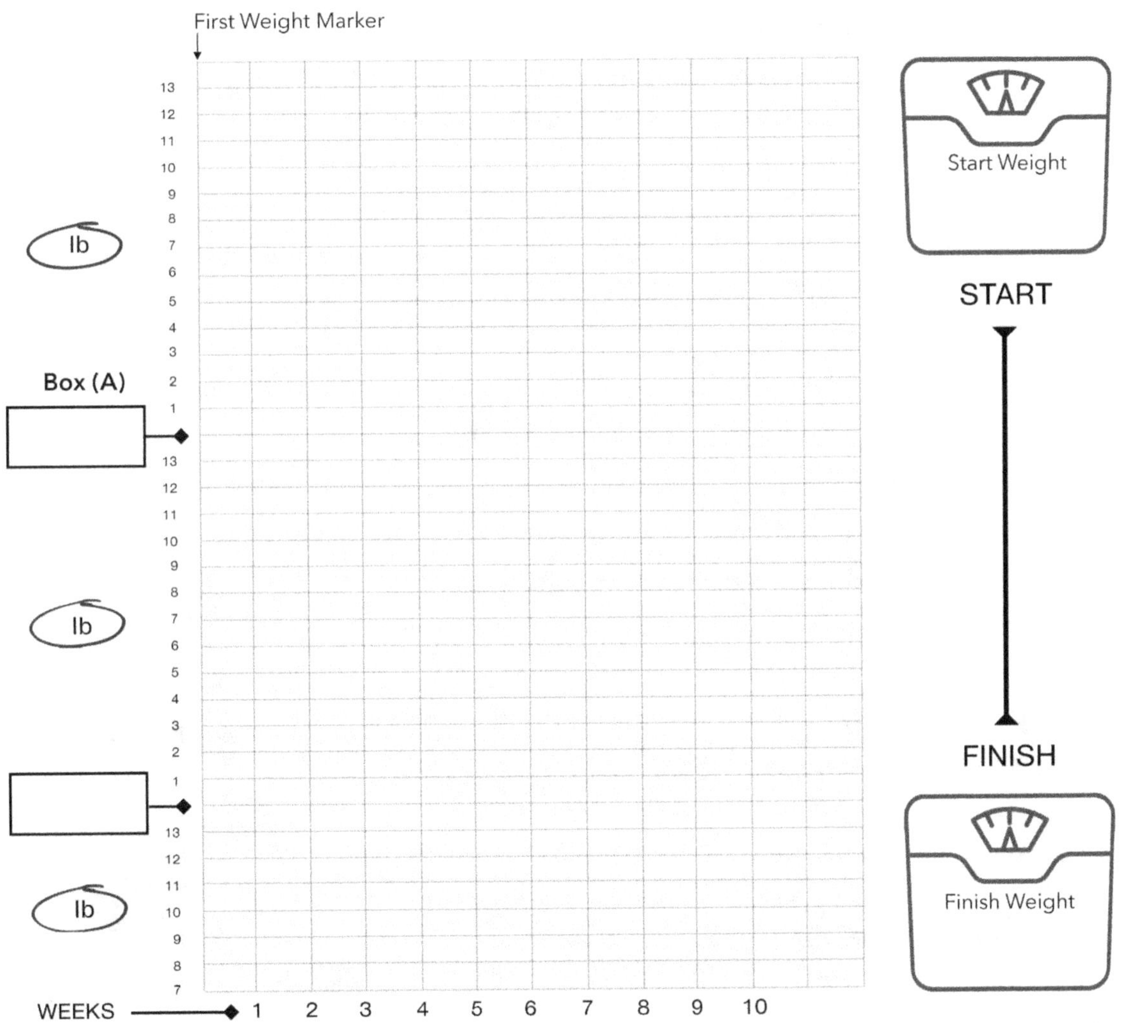

WHY DO WE NEED TO EXERCISE?

Exercising makes us fit and healthy, but not everyone has to do it!

Some people don't have to Exercise because their day to day activities are just so energy demanding, they can eat as much and as often as they like and look pretty fit, trim and healthy. These individuals have found their body balance. The energy (**Calories**) they consume is equal or less to the energy (**Calories**) they burn.

These individuals are usually heavy labourers or work in the construction industry, and they are constantly using their muscles to the maximum. For the rest of us to get to the same level of energy output, we have to play sports or hit the gym and exercise!

Sometimes it's forgotten what Exercising is all about! It is often thought of as a sport people do simply for fun and to look good.   But if you really think about it, it is an essential way of life.   If your day to day living is not burning off the energy (**Calories**) you consume, then it's something you have to do to keep your body balanced. And if you don't, well you know what happens!

So we all agree we have to Exercise.   But the downside is, it's a very confusing world out there! And I think you know what we are talking about here!

You've seen the commercials, Facebook and Youtube videos. Skinny athletic individuals jumping around without an ounce of body fat - Selling you weight loss exercise programmes and routines.

You could say I am now that skinny athletic person - Selling you the idea of an Exercise.

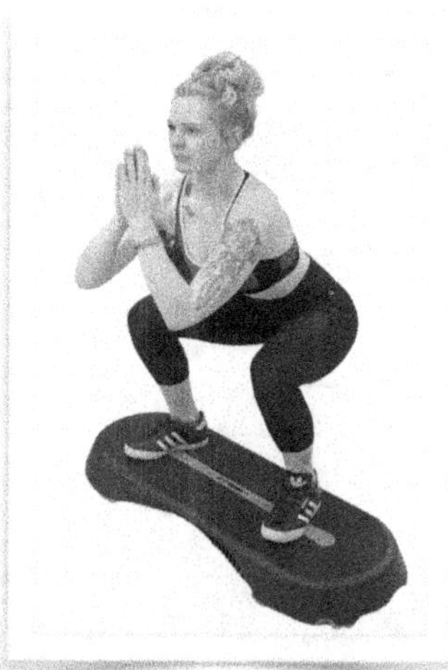

Trust me I didn't always look like this, and I certainly wasn't fit enough to perform complex Exercises.

I know what is feels like to be: 17, 16, 15, 14, 13, 12 & 11 Stone! So when it comes to Exercising for Weight loss and increased fitness - Trust me I know what I'm talking about!

EFFORT VS. REWARD

Today it seems like anyone promoting weight loss and fitness exercises are simply showing off!

The harder and more complex the exercise mechanics are, the more it seems to be pushed as a "Must do exercise". And if it's been a while since you last exercised, you may say to yourself "How can I possibly do that"?

This frustrates me greatly because the promoters of such exercises, do not take into account your age, flexibility, body shape, current stamina or fitness level. If you haven't been over active for some time, your tendons, ligaments and muscles (Including your heart) could be a little out of tune. So if you jump in at the deep end and attempt to perform a silly exercise routine, there is a chance you could do yourself some damage.

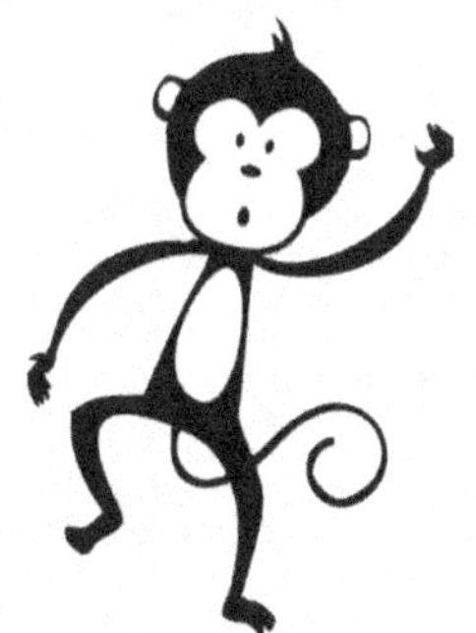

The truth is, you don't need to kill yourself by jumping around like a "**Wild Monkey**" to burn Calories. That is, not until your body is ready for it and you would enjoy it!

To start with, gentle repetition over "**Too Much Effort**" works every time. It's more productive to perform gentle Calorie burning exercises everyday, because if you are new to it all, bursts of high intensity exercises will simply leave you feeling exhausted.

High intensity and flexible challenging exercises do burn more Calories per minute, but there really isn't that much in it. And if your body isn't used to it, you will ache all over and most likely have to spend the following day laying on the sofa recovering. And who can lay on the sofa without eating a biscuit or two?

MY EXERCISE FORMULA!

I have created series of exercise plans that are designed to cater for all levels of fitness, stamina and flexibility. They work brilliantly because you get to choose the exercises that are right for you and your body type.

When I first started exercising to speed up my weight loss, I did too much too soon! I felt exhausted and repeating the process was far from my mind…!   I soon learnt how to exercise with the **RIGHT** movements for my body type. When I lost more weight and my stamina increased, I upped my game and did more. It's a wonderful catch 22…!

To save you time and increase your chances of building exercise into your life, I have created Exercise Plans that are just right for You. The best start is the right start with the right Exercises.

A video walk through for each Exercise - **and who should be doing it** - can be found on my website.

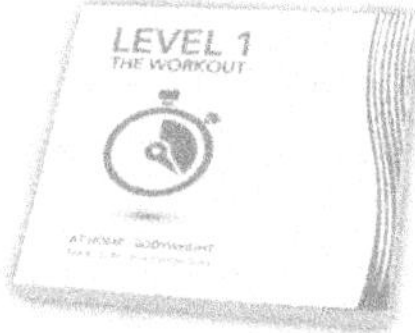

- **Level 1** - At Home, Bodyweight Exercises
- **Level 2** - At Home, Bodyweight Exercises
- **Level 3** - At Home, Bodyweight Exercises

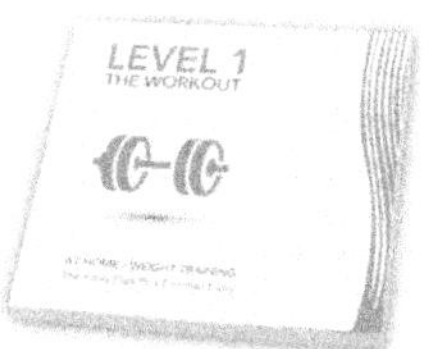

- **Level 1** - At Home, Workout With Weights
- **Level 2** - At Home, Workout With Weights
- **Level 3** - At Home, Workout With Weights

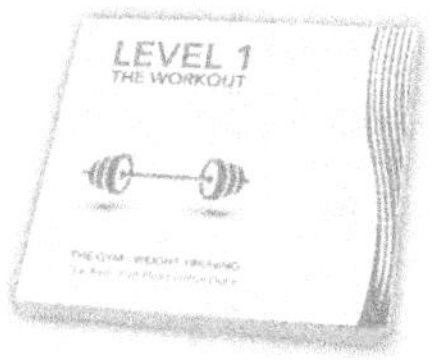

- **Level 1** - In the Gym, Bodyweight, Weights
- **Level 2** - In the Gym, Bodyweight, Weights
- **Level 3** - In the Gym, Bodyweight, Weights

When ordering these Exercise Plans/Diaries you can choose your own fun cover design. For more information please visit my website. www.thebodyplanplus.com